YOU *CAN* UNDERSTAND, TREAT, AND COPE WITH CFS

Tragically, the tormenting exhaustion and painful debilitation of chronic fatigue syndrome does not stop with the sufferer. A disease that not only invades but envelops, CFS has paralyzing symptoms that can affect the entire family, stretching the family finances—and the bonds of love—to the breaking point.

Yet, the lives and relationships of CFS sufferers *can* be healed—even as they wait for a cure to be found for this insidious disease.

Drawn from the challenges and triumphs posed by Gregg Fisher's own seven-year struggle with CFS, and culled from the findings of the most respected medical authorities in the field, this timely and compassionate guide empowers CFS sufferers and those who love them to:

- Strengthen support systems while allowing the patient to heal
- Maintain financial security and well-being no matter how prolonged the illness
- Seek out the treatments that can bolster the immune system without depleting morale
- Move beyond the grief, guilt, and anger that isolate CFS victims in their pain
- And, most of all, live each day as fully as they possibly can.

PRAISE FOR *CHRONIC FATIGUE SYNDROME*

"Inspiring . . . down-to-earth, practical, and informative. Now there's help for all who suffer from this devastating—and elusive—illness."
—MICHAEL KRAUSS, creator and executive producer, and JOAN LUNDEN, host of "Mother's Day"

"*Chronic Fatigue Syndrome* by Gregg Fisher is an intelligent account of his personal struggle and a good source of information on CFS."
—CFS Support Group Newsletter, Seattle, Washington

"*Chronic Fatigue Syndrome* is excellent—and Gregg Fisher's courage and strength are commendable."
—Wendy Cassel, R.N., California Support Group Leader

"All CFS patients should read this book. It is very beneficial and means so much to CFS patients."
—Judy Basso, President, Minnesota CEBV Association

ABOUT THE AUTHOR

Gregg Charles Fisher earned a degree in biology with a minor in chemistry from The King's College, New York, and took graduate courses in physiology and biochemistry at Rutgers University. He was attending Trinity Evangelical Divinity School when both he and his wife became ill with chronic fatigue syndrome.

CHRONIC FATIGUE SYNDROME

A Victim's Guide to Understanding, Treating and Coping With This Debilitating Illness

GREGG CHARLES FISHER

with STEPHEN E. STRAUS, M.D.;
JANET DALE, R.N.; PAUL R. CHENEY, M.D., Ph.D.;
and JAMES M. OLESKE, M.D.

A Revised and Updated Edition of
WAITING TO LIVE

WARNER BOOKS

A Time Warner Company

This book was previously published under the title *Waiting To Live*.

The information presented in this book is designed to help you better understand and cope with chronic fatigue syndrome. While this book can be a valuable addition to your doctor's advice, it is intended for your use under his or her care and direction. The author and publisher disclaim any responsibility for any adverse effects resulting from the information contained herein.

Revised and updated edition Copyright © 1989 by Gregg Charles Fisher

Copyright © 1987 by MONTCO
All rights reserved.
Warner Books, Inc., 666 Fifth Avenue, New York, NY 10103

A Time Warner Company

Printed in the United States of America
First Printing: February 1989
10 9 8 7 6 5

Library of Congress Cataloging-in-Publication Data

Fisher, Gregg Charles.
  Chronic fatigue syndrome.

  "A revised and updated edition of Waiting to live."
  Bibliography: p.
  Includes index.
  1. Chronic fatigue syndrome.   I. Straus, Stephen E.
II. Title.
RB150.F37F57   1989   616.85′28   88-33765
ISBN 0-446-39004-6 (pbk.) (U.S.A.)
      0-446-39005-4 (pbk.) (Canada)

Designed By Giorgetta Bell McRee

*This book is lovingly dedicated
to my precious Shawn,
the woman who is
my wife and my life,*

and

to

*Mary, Bernard, Caren, and Eric,
my dearly loved family:
no one embodies the true measure
of love more than you.*

CONTENTS

FOREWORD

Modern medicine has given us an air of invulnerability. Day after day, the media bring us news of the latest "wonder drug" or miracle cure. The post–World War II generation has never known the summer scourges of polio nor the mass quarantines of tuberculosis. Our concerns are the ills of advancing age: cancer, stroke, heart attacks.

Small wonder that the chronically ill are studiously ignored by the chronically well, particularly those in the prime of life. The social isolation can add an intolerable burden to an already limited life-style. Fortunately, the recent political mobilization of the physically challenged has resulted in greater accessibility to transportation and public facilities. Still, the United States is one of the few industrialized nations without a national health plan, so health costs that extend for decades keep most of the chronically ill well below the federal poverty level. The social services that might lighten the burden are all too often inaccessible to those most in need. The very effort to maintain life and limb often precludes the nourishment of heart and soul. New relationships are forestalled and existing ones are strained, often to the breaking point.

The author of this book has been faced with this type of

crisis. Taken ill while still in graduate school, trying to maintain and nurture a relationship with his future wife, he was faced with uncertain prospects of health, career, finances, and family. Many of us who have faced similar situations have had no guidance on how to proceed with our lives, or how to view our cloudy futures. This book is the very personal story of one man's journey into night. It's a saga of bewilderment, faith, despair, and hope. As with all stories of chronic illness, it's a work still in progress, but it has some wonderful lessons to teach and may serve as a wellspring of inspiration for all.

Specifically for those afflicted with this ailment, known variously as chronic fatigue syndrome, chronic Epstein-Barr virus, neuromyasthenia, myalgic encephalomyelitis, post-viral fatigue syndrome, or chronic mononucleosis, this book contains a wealth of information, in terms which are made clear to the layperson. The medical contributions are by Drs. James M. Oleske, Paul R. Cheney, Stephen E. Straus and Janet Dale, R.N., nationally recognized researchers and highly respected members of their profession.

As a fellow sufferer of this illness, and one who has spoken to hundreds of others, I endorse this book wholeheartedly, and with great affection.

ROBERT LANDAU
Support Group Leader
New Jersey CFS Association

When peace, like a river,
Attendeth my way,
When sorrows like sea-billows roll;
Whatever my lot, Thou hast
Taught me to say,
It is well, it is well
With my soul.

PREFACE

Ever since I first became ill I have recorded my experiences and reflections with the hope of someday putting them together in a book. If I had known from the outset how much effort this would cost me, I don't know if I would have attempted it. But, thanks to the help of so many others, it is done now, and I'm glad I began it.

In addition to the usual problems faced by any sufferer of a chronic illness, there is an added burden associated with chronic fatigue syndrome (CFS): it is a relatively unknown, typically unappreciated, and poorly understood disease. Although tens of thousands of people are estimated to be suffering from CFS in this country alone, and though CFS has lately been the subject of articles in medical journals, newspapers, and magazines, there is very little practical information available to help sufferers understand and cope with this terribly traumatic affliction.

My goal, then, is to supply this crucial information. But this book is not merely a compendium of impersonal information about CFS. For knowing about an illness without understanding how that illness affects the outer and inner lives of the afflicted is like knowing the statistics on hunger without understanding that people are dying of starvation. In this book I present information about CFS from my perspective as a sufferer and as the husband of a CFS sufferer as well. By showing how CFS has affected me and my family and how we have coped with it, I hope to demystify CFS for you and to suggest ways of easing the pain and frustration of living with this syndrome.

While this book was written with the help of some of the most prominent doctors involved in CFS research, I am not a doctor and cannot make a diagnosis or even recommend treatments. This book is intended solely to help you better understand and cope with CFS; you should always consult your doctor before assuming a diagnosis of CFS or trying a treatment.

The verse that opens this preface is from my favorite hymn, "It Is Well with My Soul." It expresses, in ways I never could, my greatest source of strength and support: my faith in God is my rock and my anchor. But chronic fatigue syndrome is no respecter of individual beliefs and, though I make brief references to the role faith has played in my own battle, I realize this book should not be a forum for my religious views.

What I will share with you is my personal experience and what I have learned along the way. CFS is an illness unlike any most people have ever heard of, let alone had. It's not like the flu: forty-eight hours of bed rest won't cure it; nor can it be controlled with medications. Not yet. My only escape from this viral specter that haunts my every waking moment is sleep, and yet never is rest the victor. I awake to a day as difficult as the one before it.

I have learned to hate this illness with an intensity I did not know I was capable of. But I have also learned much about CFS and about how to cope with it, insights I share with you in the pages that follow.

CHRONIC FATIGUE SYNDROME

1

Our Story

Our nightmare began in January of 1982. I was twenty-four then and attending Trinity Evangelical Divinity School, in a northern suburb of Chicago, with the dream of becoming a minister. Just three months earlier I had met Shawn, the woman who would become my wife. She was attending the same school, pursuing her master's degree in counseling and psychology. We were instantly attracted to each other, and our relationship blossomed into a lifetime commitment—one that truly tested our vow to stand by one another for better or for worse.

Our road has not taken us on the typical couple's pilgrimage toward marital bliss. For most of our dating life and all of our married life, we have both been afflicted with chronic fatigue syndrome (CFS). We are still not sure where, or even how, we contracted this illness—and we are sensible enough to avoid the question of whether one of us gave it to the other.

The first time I recall feeling ill was on a weekend trip to Minnesota. Shawn and I were visiting some of her family and friends when I became sick with what I assumed was the flu. It's not all that uncommon for students to wear themselves down until they become ill. Other than ruining my weekend, there was nothing remarkable about the experience.

I recovered enough to attend classes on Monday, and by the end of that week I was feeling much better. But about the same time, Shawn began to feel ill—and her illness did not seem like a minor case of the flu. As the days passed, it became apparent that she was suffering from something far more severe.

Every time I saw her she seemed to be dragging, as if living were a burden. She was exhausted all the time and slept constantly. She wasn't just too tired to wake up for her morning classes; she was too tired to wake up for her *evening* classes. She suffered unbearable headaches as well as a horribly painful sore throat—the kind that makes you think twice before enduring the pain of swallowing. She also found it difficult to think clearly, making studying impossible. In a word, her life was miserable.

Shawn somehow muddled through the next couple of weeks, but at great personal cost. It was obvious that her health was deteriorating. It was at this time that I too began to feel ill. My symptoms were not as severe as Shawn's, but we both realized that the symptoms were too similar to be coincidental. While we had no idea what we were suffering from, we knew it was considerably worse than the flu.

The school nurse recommended that we be tested for mononucleosis. This seemed like such a logical diagnosis, I was certain that the blood tests were merely a confirming formality. I was wrong. The results of those blood tests ushered in the most emotionally turbulent four months of my life. Shawn tested positive for mononucleosis. I did not.

All my instincts told me I had the same illness Shawn had, but the blood tests disagreed. With other possible diagnoses already ruled out, my only logical alternative at the time was to believe that I was not seriously ill. In this era of medical marvels, it never even crossed my mind that a blood test could be wrong. In my eyes, doctors were infallible. If I truly did have mononucleosis, surely they would have known.

I tried to convince myself that I was simply exhausted from my schoolwork, denying my illness in the hope that it would go away. I was so afraid of being seen as a hypochondriac that I didn't even discuss my illness with anyone else. I totally disregarded the pleas of my body for rest. As a result, my symptoms worsened.

Trapped in a bewildering world of conflicting emotions, I pushed myself to the point of exhaustion because I didn't think I had the right to be ill. Yet at the same time, I could feel my health deteriorating with each passing day. My studies suffered and my grades fell. My self-esteem was eroding as surely as my health as I blamed myself for my inability to ignore an illness that was supposed to be nothing more than minor.

Meanwhile, Shawn's health plummeted to an indescribable depth of suffering, her pain so intense that her attempts to conceal it were to no avail. Every breath required a monumental effort of will. The pain and pressure in her head were incessant. She staggered around as if in a stupor, with barely enough stamina to eat, let alone attend classes. Most of the time she slept.

But sleep only postponed the inevitable suffering until the next day. It never rejuvenated her, only numbed the pain for a few hours. This was a time of desperate need for Shawn, and there was nothing that I could do to help her. I felt like a drowning man, vainly attempting to save himself and his loved ones from perishing. I was too ill to give her the love and support she needed. I wanted to help, but my own illness frustrated all my efforts.

As the weeks passed, my own illness became impossible to ignore, yet because it paled in comparison to Shawn's suffering, I felt it no longer mattered. In my mind, my illness had become irrelevant because Shawn's was so much more severe.

As I focused on Shawn's illness to the exclusion of my own, I began to feel bitter and frustrated. I barely had enough strength to take care of myself, much less take care of her. I felt selfish for wanting her to meet my needs, and I was discouraged because there was nothing I could do to help her.

Guilt, though, is the emotion I remember most vividly from that traumatic time. I was punishing myself, trying somehow to pay for my failures. I despised myself because of my vulnerability to this illness. In point of fact I was too ill to help, but guilt blinded me, preventing me from seeing things as they really were. All I could see was how miserably I had failed.

Unable to face Shawn's pain or my own failures, I found myself withdrawing from her emotionally. She was completely unaware of the emotions I was struggling with and did not understand why I was pulling away. Never had she felt such desperate needs, and never had she felt so completely alone. These memories are still painfully vivid to both of us. To this day, Shawn is unable to remember that time without tears welling up in her eyes.

Amazingly, despite all we were enduring, one thing we never even considered was dropping out of school. At the time we had an unquestioning faith in the medical system; if no doctor told us we needed complete rest, we felt we had no choice but to struggle on. Goals like graduating on schedule seem terribly unimportant now, but at that time we had no way of knowing what we truly needed.

Also at work within us was a belief in our own invincibility. We were young, and felt anything in life could be conquered if only we were tough enough. Vulnerability was alien to us. The strong were supposed to be immune to pain and weakness; only the frail succumbed.

In the end, the innate wisdom of our bodies prevailed. We could ignore the warning signals no longer. Two weeks before the end of winter quarter we both left school. We still believed that we would soon be well, so we made arrangements with our professors to take our final exams when we returned from spring break. I remember how difficult that decision was for Shawn. Not that she was resistant to the idea of leaving; she was just too ill to think about it. Shawn's friend Carolyn and I literally had to make the decision for her. Shawn's mother came from Michigan to take her home, and I went home to New Jersey.

Often the full impact of an illness is not realized until it forces you into submission. When I went home, I collapsed from exhaustion. I hardly remember a thing from that time because I slept over sixteen hours a day, every single day for six weeks. The eight hours I wasn't sleeping, I did nothing but rest.

Shawn also slept during most of her spring break. When she awoke, it took all her strength to walk the ten feet from her bedroom to the living room couch. She was too ill to watch TV or listen to the radio. At times she even had to close the living room curtains because the sight of any activity—even of birds building their nests or squirrels foraging for food—exhausted her as if she were doing the work herself.

After six straight weeks of rest we somehow managed to drag ourselves back to school. We really believed we would be well within a few weeks and that if we could just push through for a while, we wouldn't have to miss a whole quarter. The timetable I had imposed on the next three years of my life depended on finishing all of my classes in sequence. Rather than risk my schedule, I risked my health.

Even our doctors didn't advise against returning to school. My family doctor had told me that it was possible to have mononucleosis without a positive blood test. And while he could not say I had the same illness as Shawn, he could not rule it out either.

Shawn and I were both told that these infections rarely last longer than a few months and that it would only be a matter of time until we were well. At that time, neither we nor our doctors knew that a chronic mononucleosis-like illness was even possible. As a concession to our illness, we did take a lighter load of classes, believing this would allow us a quicker recovery. In fact, returning to school completely negated the benefits of the previous six weeks of rest.

The one positive result of my return to school was that I

gained a most valuable insight. It can hurt just as much to love someone who is suffering as it does to suffer yourself. It may hurt in different ways, but the pain is no less intense.

During all the years of my illness, my greatest anguish has come not from my own illness, but as a result of Shawn's. I had built up defenses to distance myself from my own pain, but hers was like an unerring arrow that could quickly and accurately find its way into the target of my heart.

We somehow finished the quarter and went our separate ways for the summer. I had the chance to work as a youth pastor at the Calvary Evangelical Free Church back in New Jersey, a wonderful opportunity I just *couldn't* refuse. I wanted this experience so desperately that I didn't make the wise decision. Rather than trying to work sixty hours a week, I should have listened to my body and rested the entire summer.

The more I tried to be tough and push myself, the worse I felt. My situation came to a head about halfway through the summer. My throat was so swollen and painful I could hardly talk. My entire body ached. I was exhausted, dead on my feet, and finally I collapsed. I had to resign my position because I was totally incapacitated.

Fortunately, my family doctor recognized how serious—and how chronic—my condition had become, and he had heard of other doctors who were dealing with symptoms much like mine. Drs. Alan Matook and James Oleske concluded that I was suffering from an illness known at the time as chronic mononucleosis. There was no effective treatment to be offered, but what a tremendous relief it was to have a doctor identify my illness and give a name to my affliction!

Unfortunately, Shawn's experience with doctors that summer was not as good as mine. After she explained that she had been extremely ill for the last six months, her first doctor advised her to gargle with salt water and predicted she would be well in two weeks. Her next doctor had the gall to tell her that she wasn't really ill, that she was just afraid of exerting herself. Later, though he hadn't seen her in one and a half years, he informed

Social Security that she was not disabled and did not deserve benefits. Even when she sent him journal articles on CFS by respected researchers, which included descriptions of her symptoms, he refused to believe. Instead he wrote his final diagnosis in bold letters across her chart: DEPRESSION. Naturally, Shawn did not return to these doctors. In fact, she stopped seeing doctors entirely.

To this day, as a result of both our experiences, I vacillate between condemnation and praise of the medical profession. Until I saw how Shawn's doctors treated her, I did not realize how fortunate I was to have found sympathetic, informed doctors. While they might not have known what I was suffering from, they at least believed I was suffering. We cannot expect doctors to be medical encyclopedias, aware of everything there is to know in the field of medicine. Nor can we expect them not to be leery of hypochondriacal patients. But it is not too much to expect doctors to treat seriously those patients who are truly ill.

In the fall we attempted to continue our education, but in January, one year after we first became ill, we no longer had the strength to carry on. I remember coming back to my dorm room and bursting into tears. I had not defeated this illness; it had defeated me. We both withdrew from classes and returned to our parents' homes.

I do not remember very much of the next few months. That time of my life was lived unconsciously. Shawn's family, however, was quite busy. They realized that they would have to take matters into their own hands if they were to learn anything about this illness. Her father spent hours at the library doing computer searches for any reference to a chronic type of mononucleosis.

They also called doctors and research facilities looking for information. Their search eventually led them to Dr. Stephen Straus and his research coordinator, Janet Dale, of the National Institutes of Health. The NIH is our nation's research hospital, located just outside of Washington, D.C. It is a huge hospital with over fifty separate buildings and an annual budget in the billions. It also has one of the largest medical libraries in the world. People from all over the country are treated there, and since the NIH mainly researches unusual diseases, patients, who must apply to be admitted, are treated free of charge.

Our first visit lasted four days. We went through a battery of tests and were asked many questions. Dr. Straus told us that there was no cure for our illness, but that he would keep us in mind when they began researching possible treatments. Naturally we left there discouraged. We had hoped that we would hear the words "We will soon have a cure," rather than "This is just something you will have to learn to live with." Nonetheless it was a tremendous relief to learn that one of the greatest research facilities in the world not only believed in our illness, but was actually taking part in CFS research.

We became frequent visitors to the NIH, but between hospital stays we tried everything we could think of—home remedies like aloe vera juice and a bitter-tasting beef-and-wine tonic, diets, vitamin therapies, moderate exercise programs, chiropractic, and many different medications—all in the hope of finding that elusive cure. Nothing helped.

It was because I was on a special diet during one of my trips to the NIH, and had lost a considerable amount of weight, that Dr. Straus was able to feel enlarged lymph nodes in my abdomen. They were so enlarged he became alarmed and sought the opinion of another doctor. Upon examination, they both felt that, though the chance was slight, it was possible I might have cancer. They had seen five patients with the same presentation and blood results as mine. Though there were differences among us, one had developed cancer.

I was stunned. Fear and dread hung over me like a dark cloud. Despite all I had been through with CFS, I was not prepared to face the possibility of my own death. For the first time in my life I felt completely alone.

I was finally broken. I had struggled through so many emotional stages with this illness. In the beginning there was total denial. I kept pushing myself because I would not admit that I was ill. When I could no longer deny the existence of my illness, my denial had become resistance: there was not an illness in the world I couldn't master—it would be only a matter of time until I was well. But as time dragged on, resistance had slowly become desperation. Having exhausted everything that mainstream medicine had to offer, I tried anything that had even the slightest chance of being effective, no matter how outlandish the treatment.

With this terrifying news, desperation quickly slid into despair. In one fell swoop, I had to face not only the possibility that I might not get well, but the possibility that I might not live. My identity as an "ill person" was now complete. The faint flicker of hope I had for so long been fighting to keep kindled was now extinguished.

And yet, while the news was the worst I could possibly hear, I was, ironically, almost glad to hear it. At least with a diagnosis of cancer, no one could doubt that I was truly ill. After all, cancer is a relatively common disease that anyone can understand and emphathize with. Until then, I hadn't understood how desperately I needed to be believed—to hear the sympathetic words "You are truly ill," instead of the skeptical "Are you truly ill?" A part of me was willing to risk the ravages of cancer just so I would no longer have to explain my affliction or defend myself against the implication that I was lazy or crazy. I wasn't looking for pity. I just wanted the recognition and respect that other seriously ill people receive.

I was subjected to a battery of tests for cancer—blood work, X rays, ultrasound, a CAT scan, a bone scan using radioactive isotopes, and others. The most painful was a bone marrow biopsy, and I'm sure my fear that my incurable and interminable illness had spawned a more deadly disciple must have intensified the pain. I remember lying on the operating table and thinking how just two years earlier I had been perfectly healthy and looking forward to a fulfilling life. And as I endured pain greater than any I had known anyone could, I was shaken by my recognition of how radically my life had been altered by CFS. If there has been a low point in my struggle with this illness, that was it.

In the end there was no sign of cancer, but I realize now that the threat of cancer had a profound influence on my way of thinking about my life as a victim of CFS. It paved the way for my passage into the fifth and final stage of my emotional pilgrimage with CFS—acceptance. Having been faced with the threat of a terminal illness, I began to understand how precious life is, even life with a chronic illness. I realized that until a cure was found, I would have to learn to live with this illness. I could no longer avoid life and its responsibilities, waiting for a cure. I had to live now. I might not be able to live fully, but I had to make the best of the situation.

This new perspective, this determination, made possible something Shawn and I had been postponing for so long—our marriage. By then we had also learned the value of rest in harboring our most important resource, our strength. And we had built a support network of friends and family who were willing to help us over the financial hurdles. On the first of September, 1984, we were finally married, and time has proven what we then only suspected: that our emotional need for one another outweighed any possible difficulties marriage could ever present.

Our first year of marriage was, of course, more difficult than the average couple's. Between the two of us, we barely comprised one person. Taking care of our basic needs, such as cooking and cleaning, required all our strength and energy. In order to support ourselves financially, we had applied for disability benefits months before our wedding, but we were still almost a year away from receiving our first checks. Despite the generosity of the many friends and relatives who supported us during that first year, we did not have enough money to rent our own apartment. Instead we lived like nomads, staying in the homes of friends and relatives. Shawn once figured that, between moving and our trips to the NIH, we packed our bags every two weeks that year.

The reason we made so many trips to the NIH was to take part in experimental treatments. I vividly remember the last treatment I received at the NIH. My arms were jabbed with IV needles, sometimes as many as ten times in one day. As I started reacting to the treatment, I became nauseous and vomited. I broke out into a cold sweat with alternating episodes of chills and fever. My whole body ached to the point where I broke down and cried, wondering how I could possibly hope to cope with this illness when I could barely cope with a possible cure. I was afraid to continue with this treatment because of its side effects, while at the same time afraid that the drug might not take effect.

Because of their often painful side effects and uncertain results, I've never felt comfortable submitting myself to experimental treatments. But they do offer the only chance of a cure, or, at the very least, some relief, something we, like all CFS sufferers, need desperately. And so I undergo them, learning to walk a careful line between sensible optimism and naive hope. I need my optimism to maintain my determination, but frankly, I am terrified of hope, which is so easily dashed to pieces on the rocks of reality. In fact, the one time that I seriously contemplated suicide was because I let my hopes get the upper hand.

I was under the care of a physician who boasted that he knew exactly what was wrong with me and guaranteed that I would be well enough to return to school in a few short weeks. Wanting desperately to believe him, I foolishly let my guard down and allowed my hopes to soar. After a month of costly and painful tests and treatments, he casually informed me that there was nothing more he could do and would I please leave because he was expecting another patient. No apologies, no explanations.

Abandoned not only by the doctor but by my own sustaining

sense of hope, I fell into a depression—exacerbated, I suspect, by the medication he had given me—that brought me to the brink of suicide. Fortunately, I stopped taking the medication and began to recover from my depression. I was able to work through my suicidal feelings without acting upon them, but the experience has left its legacy. Whether for good or for ill, I resist opening myself up to the extremes of feeling, both other people's and my own, and I am especially cautious never to be vulnerable to the perils of unreasonable hope.

Lately our lives have been a series of trips to various doctors and hospitals. Researching our illness, undergoing treatments, and taking care of our basic needs require all of our time and strength. We are able to socialize only rarely and have been unable to return to school or to work even part-time.

But it has been interesting to be involved in the "discovery" of a disease—to have been a CFS patient when this illness had no name and was not recognized by more than a handful of physicians. Our case histories were presented before the Senate Subcommittee on Health and Human Services in an appeal for funding for CFS research. We have also participated in research to determine the efficacy of various experimental treatments.

Whatever we are forced to endure because of CFS, however an experiment may turn out, it is of some comfort to remember that no research is ever done in vain. Science does not march directly to its answers. No effort is without value if it adds to the body of knowledge. It is all a necessary part of the work of uncovering the cause of and cure for CFS. And, in fact, it is exciting to see the changes that are starting to occur.

When we first became ill, only a few doctors were aware of this syndrome and there were only vague references in the medical literature. Now, some of the most prestigious health organizations in the country, such as the NIH, the Centers for Disease Control, and the Food and Drug Administration, have recognized the legitimacy of this syndrome. Doctors all across the country are actively pursuing research and there is ongoing communication with other countries as well. Many new organizations are being formed to raise money for CFS research, and the general public is becoming increasingly aware of the problem. All of these changes can only lead to more research and an eventual cure. We can take heart knowing that it is only a matter of time until that cure is found.

In the meantime, Shawn and I strive to live each day as best we can. As difficult and painful as this illness is, we try to enjoy what life has to offer. We appreciate the simple pleasures and are grateful for the love we share with each other and with those around us.

Through the long years of this illness, we have had to struggle every day to cope with our affliction. As the years go by, we are more determined than ever to remain strong. The saying that time heals all wounds is true, not because wounds, like sand castles, wash away with the first tide but because in time you learn to survive your wounds.

Give yourself the time to learn to live with your wound. Shawn and I have managed it, and you can too. Hope comes not from seeing what is, but from dreaming of what might be.

2
Symptoms

We should never judge the validity of another person's pain based solely on whether there are observable physical findings. Nowhere is this more important to understand than with CFS. Not only is the physical distress often unobservable, it is also not the only kind of pain inflicted by a serious illness. The emotional, mental, and spiritual pain can be just as harsh.

The pain and sickness I experience is debilitating, but very little of my suffering is ever witnessed by the outside world. People don't see me when I'm having horrible days. They see me only for brief periods of time when I have rested enough to act as normally as possible. The next few days, when I am home alone, I suffer the unwitnessed consequences of that activity. Ironically, what I perceive as my noble effort to endure bravely and silently the pain of my illness, others misconstrue to mean I am not really suffering. Unfortunately, as yet, the fact that there are no laboratory tests to confirm a CFS diagnosis makes this illness one that does not lend itself to credibility. In fact, I know only a handful of people who believe without reservation in my illness. I'm afraid that many people, because of their unfamiliarity with CFS and its often unobservable symptoms, tend to see me as either a hypochondriac or a malingerer.

I realize that I have an unusual illness. My symptoms appear vague and insignificant, and I invariably look much better than I feel. From a doctor's perspective, the severity of CFS symptoms is completely out of proportion to any objective physical findings—blood tests or physical exams often don't reveal significant abnormalities. But such tests also don't reveal the devastating effects of CFS on the lives of sufferers—their loss of careers, possessions, even their loved ones. I know a woman, for example, who was so incapacitated by CFS that she had to give up her baby to be raised by her mother. I know of women whose husbands left them because CFS disrupted their marriages. Many lose high-paying jobs and must rely on disability checks that come to only a fraction of their former salary.

To keep my sanity while surrounded by so much doubt, I remind myself of two important truths I must accept. The first is that my appearance will forever make it hard for outsiders to respect the severity of my illness. The second is that there will always be people who judge with their eyes rather than with their hearts. These people understand only what they want to understand. To them, my illness will always seem more like a crutch, masking deep psychological problems, than a cry of pain caused by a very real sickness.

Most symptoms are, by nature, subjective accounts of how a person feels and are not objective proof by which to substantiate a diagnosis. And yet with CFS, symptoms so far are all we have to work with. To resolve this dilemma, and to provide some guidelines for researchers and practitioners, Dr. Gary Holmes and others have formulated what is called a case definition of CFS, published in the March 1988 issue of *Annals of Internal Medicine*.

Simplified, the definition states that a case of CFS must meet two major criteria: debilitating fatigue that does not go away with bed rest and that reduces a person's average daily activity by more than 50 percent, and also the elimination, through physical examinations, laboratory tests, and patient history, of a long list of diseases that could cause similar symptoms.

Beyond fulfilling the two major criteria, the patient must

fulfill the minor criteria by having eight or more of the following eleven symptoms: mild fever, sore throat, painful lymph nodes, unexplained generalized muscle weakness, muscle discomfort or pain, fatigue lasting more than twenty-four hours after exercise, headaches, joint pain without redness or swelling, a neuropsychologic complaint such as depression or confusion or inability to concentrate, sleep disturbance, and the original onset of symptoms developing rapidly, over a few hours or days.

In Chapter 4, "Diagnosis," I will discuss in more detail how these criteria are applied. In this chapter, I describe the symptoms most frequently experienced with CFS, starting with the most common ones. Much of what I describe is based on my own experience, so it's important to remember that no one has every symptom. Some people experience a particular symptom all the time, while others experience it intermittently. Some symptoms occur cyclically, for instance one week out of every month, while others occur randomly. The severity of the symptoms varies from person to person. Many people with CFS are totally disabled, while others are merely annoyed. Typically, the severity of a symptom will be exacerbated by an increase in activity—the more you do, the worse you feel. Remember also that some of the symptoms I describe may not sound very debilitating. In fact, at one time or another, almost everyone experiences such symptoms as fatigue or headaches. However, degree is the key word here: CFS fatigue is to end-of-the-day tiredness what lightning is to a spark.

There is one more thing I want to warn you about before I describe the symptoms of CFS. It seems a part of human nature to compare ourselves with others (the first thing a student does when he gets a test back is to compare his grade with the person sitting next to him). It can be terribly self-destructive to do this with an illness. Other people's symptoms are not a yardstick by which to measure the severity of your own illness. You can't really know how other people are feeling even if they describe their symptoms. So please don't use my experience in an attempt to validate your own. Knowing that you hurt is all that is required to validate what you feel. When you understand this you free yourself to acknowledge your own pain without feeling guilty that others may be more ill—the trap I at first fell into when Shawn seemed so much sicker than I did.

Knowing that there are others whose suffering is similar to mine gives me strength. If you are a victim of CFS, you can also have the strength that comes from knowing that you are not suffering alone. But only you know how debilitating your illness is. You should not be intimidated by what may seem like a more severe illness, nor should you trivialize the experience of someone who doesn't seem as ill as you. If you are in pain, all that matters is that you hurt.

FATIGUE

This is by far the most common symptom experienced by people with CFS. Unfortunately, fatigue is such a common condition for the average American that our complaints are often dismissed out of hand as mere whining. But fatigue of CFS can't be compared to the fatigue of a healthy person. It transcends anything I had ever experienced before I became ill.

Not one moment goes by that I don't feel exhausted. I often feel like the Titan Atlas holding up the world—except that rather than easily bearing its enormous weight, I am weakly crushed beneath it. And my fatigue is not only physical. The tremendous mental, emotional, and spiritual drain of this illness is wearying beyond imagination.

I yearn for the simple pleasure of restful and refreshing sleep. Instead, though I am forced to rest and sleep a full two-thirds of my life, I feel just as exhausted when I wake up in the morning as I did when I went to bed. It is misery to go through each day as exhausted as the day before, to go to sleep every night knowing I am not going to feel rejuvenated when I awake, to regard my bed as a prison because that is where I am sentenced to spend most of my life.

To an outsider trying to understand why my fatigue is so debilitating, I can only liken it to the Chinese water torture. One day of fatigue, like one drop of water, does not seem terribly tormenting. But the unending presence of fatigue, like the incessant flow of water drops, is torturous. Anyone can withstand the strain of exhaustion for one day, but when that day stretches out into years, the strain can feel intolerable. There is no surrender, though, for my very survival depends upon withstanding that strain.

Some people with this illness do have occasional respites from their fatigue. For them, this symptom is intermittent rather than incessant. Others are completely bedridden. Between these two extremes are the rest of us, too exhausted to do most of the things we'd like to in our lives.

There is a tendency for some people with this illness to feel different levels of fatigue at different times of the day. For instance, they may feel a little less tired in the morning. The only change I experience with this symptom is when it worsens, usually following activity.

I cope with my fatigue by acceding to its demands of rest, rest, and more rest. I don't like this new life-style that has been forced upon me, but I have adjusted to it as a prisoner adjusts to his jail cell. I accept its stringent requirements because I have no other choice. Resting does not eliminate fatigue, but it does prevent me from feeling worse, and that is no small accomplishment. To someone with CFS, not feeling worse often seems like the next best thing to being cured.

There is nothing that I do without first weighing the benefits against the detriments, for there is nothing that I do that is not detrimental to one degree or another. I prioritize, eliminating from my schedule activities that require the most amount of strength while giving the least reward, because I pay for every activity with the currency of exhaustion.

In the beginning, I was very resistant to this new life-style. I believed that letting CFS dictate my activities was tantamount to cowardly surrender. I thought that if I could be tough enough and persistent enough, I would conquer this illness. After years of making myself worse by foolishly trying to beat an unbeatable foe, I realized I was mistaking intelligence for cowardice. Mentally and emotionally I've neither given up nor given in. At least for now, however, I have surrendered to the absolute necessity of giving in physically. Only by resting do I have a chance of coping with this illness.

MALAISE

When I'm grocery shopping I frequently have to sit down right in the middle of the store, not only because I am physically tired but because malaise makes simple mental tasks, such as choosing between two products, draining to the point of exhaustion. It can also make everyday tasks like phone calls seem complicated and overwhelming.

Malaise is my most devastating symptom. The word means ''ill feeling''—a terribly inadequate definition for such a woeful beast. But how do I describe my worst nightmare? How can I be objective about something that I loathe?

When I describe this symptom to people who have CFS, I call it ''my dazed, CFS feeling.'' They usually know immediately what I'm referring to. But that doesn't explain much to someone unfamiliar with CFS. If I said I was sick to my stomach, most people would understand exactly what I meant. But how do I tell you what it's like to be sick to my brain? I don't mean a headache, I mean a brainache!

My mind refuses to function properly, but it's not just an inability to think clearly. It's a pressure in my head that forces me to focus inward on my illness, making me unable to interact with the rest of the world. It's as if a fence has been placed between me and the world, keeping it tantalizingly close yet hopelessly out of reach. Even my senses are affected. Nothing tastes, feels, smells, sounds, or looks as good as it did before, for nothing penetrates the malaise without being filtered and distorted.

Sometimes even emotions can't breach these prison walls. I feel as if I exist on a flat, emotionless plain with none of the peaks or valleys of normal experience. There are other times, though, when just the negative emotions come through. My anger, frustration, and despair overwhelm me and I long to be back in the emotionless state.

The worst aspect of malaise is that it interferes with my ability to cope with my illness. How can I handle the tremendous burdens CFS imposes when malaise robs me of the emotional and mental tools needed to do exactly that? Though I feel like a prisoner of my own mind, I also feel surgically removed from it. In one sense I am locked in, but in another I am locked out.

Obviously, I have not found any quick or easy solutions to this dilemma that haunts me. What I *have* learned is that there is a correlation between an increase in my activity and an increase in my malaise, so resting at least helps prevent a worsening of this symptom. If an effective treatment for CFS ever comes along, I'll know it by its ability to clear my hated malaise.

SORE THROAT

A sore throat is another common symptom of CFS. While mine is obviously painful, it is not constant and unrelenting the way my fatigue and malaise are. Another difference is that my malaise and fatigue don't become more severe until hours after an activity, while my sore throat gets worse almost immediately.

It is my first indication that I have been pushing myself too hard.

This sore throat is not like those I experienced before I became ill. It is a much duller ache. While the pain can radiate all the way up to my ears and head, it seems to start much deeper down in the throat. The pain and swelling may be centered near the vocal cords, too deep to be noticed by the average doctor using a tongue depressor. If your throat really hurts, you may want to go to an ear, nose, and throat specialist (ENT). They have the proper instruments to examine your throat. Many times, only an ENT specialist will be able to notice any appreciable swelling or irritation.

I have heard of some people who have such painful sore throats that they actually are prevented from swallowing. Mine has never been that severe, but it still interferes with the already difficult task of communicating with other people. If the malaise doesn't prevent me from talking, the sore throat will.

The worst aspect of a sore throat is, obviously, that it hurts. Pain is not easily ignored. It seems to reach out and grab me and say, "Pay attention!" and I have no choice but to do just that. Pain doesn't let go until it is gone.

Unfortunately, I know of nothing to relieve the pain. Resting is preventive medicine, and gargling with warm salt water may bring temporary relief. Shawn, whose sore throat is constant and much more severe than mine, has discovered what she says is the only truly effective "treatment" for the temporary (albeit fattening) relief of her sore throat—milk shakes! Her treatment may not be sanctioned by the medical profession, but it does seem to help. And besides, what other medicine can you look forward to taking?

FEVER

Fever is one of the few symptoms of CFS that is objectively measurable, yet while most patients will complain of feeling feverish, few will actually demonstrate a very high temperature. In fact, the entire time I have had CFS I have felt feverish, yet my temperature has rarely risen to over 100 degrees. From a patient's perspective, a symptom is a subjective impression, not an objective fact. You need not have an inordinately high temperature to validate your feverish feeling.

Most temperature readings are taken orally, and while this may be easiest, it is not the most accurate. The actual body temperature may be higher or lower than what the thermometer indicates.

Also, the temperature reading of 98.6 degrees Fahrenheit that we call normal is only an average. Everyone's "thermostat" is set a little bit differently; normal for many people may be a little higher or a little lower. A temperature reading of 99 degrees may actually indicate a fever in someone who typically has a lower body temperature.

I have not noticed any significant fluctuation in my feverishness during the course of a day. It never becomes very severe, but it never goes away. There are people with CFS, however, who do feel more feverish depending on the time of day. Since this symptom is less severe than many of my others, it is difficult for me to discern exactly how it affects me. I know that it contributes to the flulike feeling that I associate with CFS, but it is not particularly devastating. I have not found anything that significantly alleviates this symptom beyond cold compresses on the head and aspirin.

DEPRESSION

As a CFS sufferer, I have discovered that this symptom has a physical as well as a psychological dimension. CFS has manifested itself physically by debilitating me. It has *depressed* me in the very literal sense that it has severely limited my strength and activity.

Of course the constant pain and frustration of a chronic illness like CFS can have a profound emotional impact on a sufferer, resulting in depression. Depression is not something that you should allow to go untreated. It is very dangerous when it is suppressed and allowed to grow. It prevents clear and rational thinking, causing bitterness, self-absorption, and emotional instability. This can destroy your chances of coping with your illness.

LYMPHADENOPATHY

Lymphadenopathy is the technical term for enlarged lymph nodes, a very common symptom of many diseases, including CFS. Lymph nodes are found throughout the body and function as a clearinghouse for the lymphatic system. This veinlike circulatory system collects the fluids, proteins, and foreign substances that accumulate between the cells of the body, and it recycles anything that can be reused.

Lymph nodes help to filter out and dispose of undesirable matter, such as bacteria or refuse. They are also the site where many of the white blood cells of the immune system are stored and matured. Therefore, enlarged or tender lymph nodes frequently indicate that the body is actively fighting an infection.

Even though lymph nodes are found throughout the entire body, your doctor will probably examine three main areas: the neck, under the arms, and the abdomen. While enlarged lymph nodes are a normal and typically benign consequence of having certain infections, they should always be examined by a physician. Though it is a rare occurrence with CFS, there are certain types of cancers, called lymphomas, that are associated with the lymphatic system.

The effect of enlarged lymph nodes is usually not serious, but can cause some pain and discomfort. Patients with CFS generally do not have substantial enlargement of lymph nodes, but rather intermittent node tenderness.

HEADACHES

Headaches are miserable. Everybody hates a headache. What other relatively minor affliction is single-handedly capable of supporting its own multimillion-dollar-a-year drug industry? (Headaches are to the aspirin industry what taxes are to politicians: something they publicly disdain but are privately grateful for.)

The problem is that you can't ignore a headache. It may be minor compared to other ailments, but it is major in its ability to prevent you from doing or thinking about anything else. You just can't be yourself until it is gone. This seems especially true of CFS headaches—maybe because they come in tandem with so many other horrible symptoms.

Fortunately, I don't have these headaches all the time. Like many other symptoms of this illness, my headache is worse when I have been active. Some people find relief with aspirin or other analgesics. I've tried most of the major pain relievers, but the only way I can relieve a headache is to turn out all the lights and lie down. Usually within a couple of hours the headache is gone.

JOINT PAIN

As anyone confined to a wheelchair can attest, it isn't easy to be immobile in a mobile society. Our world isn't geared to accommodate those who can't keep up with its fast and frenzied pace. The joint pain that strikes many people with CFS, while varying in intensity and not always constant, can prevent you from doing just that.

Joint pain affects many different areas of the body, including the knees, ankles, fingers, wrists, elbows, shoulders, and hips. Some people are so debilitated they are actually confined to a wheelchair. Others are able to get around by using a cane, while many are just not able to move as easily as they used to.

Many people notice that their joint pain is worse during a flare-up of their illness or following increased activity. For some this symptom ebbs and flows for no apparent reason. Most people only experience this pain intermittently. During those times, they try to limit their activities, but if the pain strikes areas such as the arms or hands, simple tasks like cooking or cleaning can become a study in pain and frustration.

I consider myself quite fortunate because I have had only one experience with severe joint pain since I became ill. During a particularly bad flare-up of my illness, I started noticing some pain in my knees. It wasn't a sharp pain, more of a dull ache. I noticed it especially when I pushed the clutch down in our car. The pain became so intense, driving became impossible. I couldn't even walk a few short steps. I went to see an orthopedist, but he could find nothing physically wrong with my knees. He did fit me for braces, which enabled me to support myself with less pain and effort.

After about four to six weeks the pain was suddenly gone. Not coincidentally, the relief coincided with the end of the general flare-up of my illness. I still don't know why I had that experience then; I've had many other severe flare-ups with no sign of joint pain.

There seem to be a thousand times more questions than answers with this illness and even fewer methods of relief. You might try commercial pain relievers, similar to arthritis medications. If the pain becomes so severe that you can't even walk, ask your doctor for some prescription-strength medicine. If walking is difficult, don't be embarrassed to use a cane.

INABILITY TO THINK CLEARLY

At first glance, this must seem like a terribly unremarkable symptom and very similar to malaise. They are similar in that both affect the mind, but they don't always go hand in hand. In my experience, this symptom is different from malaise because it does not involve a sick, dazed, clouded feeling. Rather, it reflects confusion, impairing the ability to reason abstractly.

I am most aware of this symptom when I am attempting to do some simple mental task. When reading, I will suddenly be unable to recall a single word I've just read. I can write a sentence and be unsure if what I've just written makes a bit of sense. I can listen to people speak and not understand what they are saying, as if they're speaking at 78 rpm but I'm listening at 33⅓.

My wife is most affected by this symptom when she tries to drive. The roar of a passing truck, the changing traffic lights, the hubbub of pedestrians on the street all bewilder her, making the safe operation of a car impossible. Even the simple act of crossing the street can be perplexing and mystifying.

Inability to think clearly can make a CFS patient appear slow or even mentally impaired. This is particularly distressful for people with CFS because many of them are very intelligent people. Some of them are students who find themselves unable to complete their assignments or do well on tests. Others are involved in business and can no longer keep up with their colleagues. As with malaise, I have not found any relief for this symptom.

The symptoms described above are considered the standards of CFS. By that I mean that they are the ones most frequently experienced. The symptoms that follow are not as universally experienced. I have experienced some of them only once or twice and others not at all. But they are no less important or indicative of the presence of CFS, just a little less common.

WEIGHT LOSS

Weight loss, while a symptom of CFS, has the distinction of being one of the few symptoms that does not appear to be directly caused by the illness. It may be that some people with CFS experience weight loss simply because they are too exhausted to prepare nutritious meals. Maybe their desire for food, like their desire for everything else, is suppressed by their illness. Perhaps they are so emotionally and physically depressed that they don't care enough about themselves to eat properly.

My only experience with weight loss came from trying "health conscious" diets, every one of them guaranteed to make me healthy as an ox. All I did was lose weight that, being thin already, I could ill afford to lose. If you're interested in trying a diet, you might want to discuss it first with a nutritionist or your doctor.

If you find you are losing weight unaccountably, take a step back and try to determine the cause. If your desire for food is gone because nothing tastes good anymore, you have to begin regarding your food as you would medicine. It may not taste very good, but it is terribly important for your health.

SKIN RASHES

I have experienced skin rashes only twice during my illness. The first time was when I went to see a doctor only a month after I became ill. Baffled by my early symptoms of fatigue and malaise, he didn't know what else to do for me and prescribed penicillin. Within a day, I had broken out into hives all over my body. I have since learned that hives are a classic reaction when someone with infectious mononucleosis is given penicillin.

The second time I had a skin rash was when I was a patient in an experimental drug therapy program at the National Institutes of Health. They were trying to determine the efficacy of acyclovir on CFS. I broke out in welts, mostly on my abdomen. They were much larger but less numerous than the hives I had before. In both cases, my rashes were in response to drug treatments. However, some people experience rashes even though they are not on any medication.

Since rashes are a common allergic reaction, it's possible that a patient's allergies are interacting with the illness. There does not seem to be one specific rash associated with CFS. Therefore, the illness may be unmasking preexisting allergic conditions that only now show themselves in the form of a rash. Ask your doctor or dermatologist for medication that can relieve this symptom.

MEMORY LOSS

I personally find this symptom terribly disturbing (but I can't remember why)!

I used to pride myself on my memory. In fact, it replaced diligent study as my principal means of getting through school. Now, I have such a terrible memory that I sometimes don't even bother trying.

Some people with CFS are affected more severely in their short-term memory. They can't remember where they just put something or what they are supposed to do the next hour. I have more difficulty with my long-term memory. I have trouble remembering the names of people that I have known for a long time.

The years since I've been ill are especially blurry. Part of the problem may lie in the fact that nothing terribly remarkable happens in my life anymore. Nothing changes, not even the symptoms of my illness. While healthy people's lives have memorable highs and lows, mine is static and stationary and lacking in memorable experiences.

Memory loss is another neurological symptom of CFS that may have a physiological component as well as a psychological one. Either way, I have unfortunately found nothing that helps alleviate this symptom.

PERSONALITY CHANGES

Personality changes are practically synonymous with CFS. I have become very moody since I became ill. If I am not angry, I am sad. If I am not frustrated, I am depressed. I have so many mood swings that I hardly remember what the old me was like.

What's happening is that my personality is reflecting whatever emotion I happen to be struggling with at the time. This disease has worn me down so completely that I have neither the strength nor the desire to put up facades. With only enough strength to survive each day, one day at a time, there is no energy left over for masking my emotions.

This seems to me to be a natural consequence of living with such a taxing chronic illness. Beyond psychiatric intervention should your mood swings get out of hand, I can only recommend that you help the people around you to understand what you are going through so they can be patient and compassionate.

SLEEP DISTURBANCE

It is not easy falling asleep when your throat hurts, your head is splitting, and your joints are aching. It is quite easy to understand, then, that sleep, even for people as exhausted as we are, might not be easily achieved. But the inability to fall asleep is only part of what this symptom entails.

Even if sleep finally comes, there is no guarantee that it will be long or restful. I have often slept for twelve hours or more, only to wake up feeling much sicker than I did the night before. I believe part of the reason is that I did not get a good night's sleep. Sometimes I wake up two or three times during the night, totally disoriented. Other nights I toss and turn so much, I use more energy than I gain.

When sleep is elusive, many people take sleeping pills. I have a prescription for a very mild sedative for those nights when I am too exhausted to sleep yet sleep is the only remedy for that exhaustion. I dislike the addictive property of sleeping pills, so I am very careful and use them only about ten times a year.

If you push yourself beyond your limits, allowing your body to rest only when you sleep, you should consider reevaluating your priorities and slowing down. The more you rest during the day, the less critical sleep will be at night.

IRRITABILITY

I had trouble deciding whether or not this symptom actually deserved a heading of its own. It could easily be included under personality changes and still be explained fairly well. I realized in the end that this is such a common emotion among patients with CFS that it merits special recognition.

Like my mood swings, irritability is dictated totally by my illness. Unfortunately, it is dictated almost constantly. I marvel at the times I am *not* irritable rather than at the times I am.

Irritability is always just below the surface, ready to explode and spew forth its poison. Healthy people normally maintain a buffer zone that allows them to let life's little annoyances slide off their backs. But weakness and frustration with my illness have gotten the better of my patience. I feel like a lion on the prowl, waiting for some poor unsuspecting person to say the wrong thing or, better yet, give me the wrong look. You know the look I mean, the one that tells you that no matter what they say, they really don't believe in your illness. In the beginning, I had better control over my emotions, and I said nothing. Today, the person who commits so egregious an error receives the full brunt of my pent-up frustrations.

NIGHT SWEATS

While night sweats are not as debilitating as most of the other symptoms, they are yet another peculiar piece in the CFS puzzle. I will sometimes suddenly awake to find myself dripping with perspiration, as if I had run a marathon in my sleep.

Night sweats occur randomly and without warning, and so far I have been unable to identify the cause. Fortunately, they are nothing to be overly concerned about. Other than feeling uncomfortable, night sweats are quite painless.

CHEST PAINS

I have never experienced this symptom, but any pain that might be associated with the heart should not be dismissed lightly. Some people with CFS experience a tightening around the chest. Some also experience palpitations, or a racing heart. Although there are no studies correlating CFS with heart problems, remember that you don't need to have CFS to have heart problems. You can have two totally unrelated ailments. So please go to your physician immediately when you experience any type of heart or chest pains. Don't dismiss chest pains simply because you have had them before or because you think they are merely another symptom of this syndrome. Chest pains always need further evaluation.

I have discussed the major and most common symptoms associated with CFS, but they are not the only ones. The following is a list of other symptoms that have been reported in the literature on CFS or that I have heard about from various CFS sufferers.

Dizziness
Disorientation
Odd skin sensations
Intolerance of temperature extremes
Swelling of the hands
Loss of muscle coorination
Weakness

Numbness and lack of feeling
Digestive problems
Intolerance of alcohol
Sensitivity to light and noise
Chills
Splenomegaly (enlarged spleen)
Hepatomegaly (enlarged liver)
Swelling of the eyelids
Nausea
Diarrhea
Tinnitus (ringing of the ears)
Earaches
Bladder problems
Muscle pain
Excessive sleep
Balance problems
Shortness of breath
Abdominal cramping

It is important to emphasize here that not only enlarged lymph nodes or chest pains, but any serious symptom should be reported to a doctor. CFS patients sometimes attribute everything they feel to CFS. This is potentially dangerous because we are still capable of developing other medical problems, mild or serious, that should not be ignored.

A discussion of CFS symptoms would not be complete if I didn't share an observation about the word *complaint*, a word I often use in discussing these symptoms. One of its dictionary definitions is "a bodily ailment or injury," which is how I mean it when I use it in reference to symptoms. But it's an easy word to misconstrue—and that makes it an interesting analog for my illness. Anyone who accepts the reality of CFS will understand what I mean by *complaint*. A skeptic will hear it as a whine, a gripe. As with so much in illness, understanding rests on belief.

3

Understanding Your Illness

With an illness like CFS, whose history is so filled with confusion and doubt, gaining a clear understanding of what your illness is—and is not—becomes your obligation as a CFS patient. I have heard heartbreaking stories of people who wandered from doctor to doctor, desperate to find someone to identify the cause of their suffering, or who spent their precious strength proving their sanity to skeptical psychiatrists when they should have been pursuing treatment for their very real illness.

The benefit of understanding your illness is not limited to avoiding the problems that others have been through. Only by understanding your illness can you gain the wisdom you need to confidently take responsibility for your own health and welfare—a responsibility that should never be abdicated to anyone, not even to a caring doctor or a loving friend.

Not that I suggest you refuse the help of a loved one or that you spurn a competent doctor's advice. On the contrary, no other illness forces a person to rely more heavily on the help and support of others. But only you know the specific burdens you are dealing with; only you can decide how best to cope with those burdens.

If you had an ailment that a doctor could remove surgically or cure with drugs, you might be able to relinquish your responsibility for self-determination. But CFS is a perplexing disease that often takes doctors beyond their own knowledge and understanding into areas where they may be no more qualified than you to make decisions that will affect your life. Often a doctor will be able to offer you options—some potentially helpful therapy or treatment, perhaps even the chance to try an experimental drug—but will have no way of predicting the results, or even of guaranteeing that you won't come to some further harm. Only you can make a decision like that, and to do it intelligently you need to understand your illness first.

This proposal may be frightening to some of you. It is much easier and less intimidating to leave the difficult decisions to someone else. And frankly, not all of us are in the habit of studying complicated scientific concepts. But often what is easiest is not what is best. Because I try to learn all I can about my illness, I am in a position to work side by side with my doctors, they relying on me for information as much as I rely on them.

Most important of all, never stop striving to learn more about your illness. I intend this book as a base, a starting point, toward a better understanding of CFS, but you should not limit your understanding only to what I have written. Even as I write, much of this information is on its way to being out of date; new and important information, I'm glad to say, is constantly being discovered about viral illnesses and the immune system in general and about CFS in particular.

There are several organizations that function as clearinghouses for new information (see Appendix C); they can help you obtain copies of any relevant articles pertaining to CFS. If you don't understand some of the technical language in the articles, ask your doctor for a translation. If your doctor refuses to do so simple and important a service, find another doctor.

You may feel overwhelmed by the immense challenge of being fully responsible for your health. Please understand that what I am advising is a process, not an end unto itself. I am urging that you slowly but surely increase your understanding of this syndrome and of how it specifically affects your life. As your understanding increases, so will your confidence.

I've tried to make the science in this chapter easy to understand, but probably some of you will find parts of it rough going. Don't worry. Read as much of each section as you can digest at one time. I've organized each section with the general, and most important, information first and the more technical material after that. If you get stuck, go on to the next section, where you'll find more information that will be useful to you. Perhaps later, when you have a clearer picture of what the science is about, you will go back and fill in the pieces you've missed.

CFS, MONO, AND ME

Like many people with chronic fatigue syndrome, I think of my illness as mononucleosis that never went away. The reason being, I'm unable to determine when my mononucleosis stopped and my CFS started. (Actually, it's never been proved that my CFS started with a bout of mono, but since Shawn and I got sick at the same time, and her blood work confirmed that she had mono, and since it's possible to have mono and still have a negative monospot test as I did, I'm 95 percent sure that mine started with mono too.)

I know that many doctors believe that for a mononucleosis-like illness to be considered CFS, it must first have persisted for at least half a year. From my perspective, however, nothing terribly dramatic happened on the 183rd day of my illness. I felt just as miserable on that day as I did the day before. After all, the two illnesses are so similar symptomatically that from a patient's point of view, they may be virtually indistinguishable.

In fact, in the past, episodes of similar fatigue syndromes were usually referred to in the medical literature as chronic mononucleosis. In recent years, however, doctors and patients have begun to recognize the importance of distinguishing between these two illnesses.

One reason for establishing a unique identity for CFS, as Dr. Holmes and his colleagues have done by devising a case definition for CFS (see Chapters 2 and 4), is to prevent the pain and frustration of a succession of misdiagnoses, ranging from lupus to AIDS. Many CFS patients are unable to trace the onset of their illness to an initial episode of mononucleosis. If this illness continued to be called chronic mononucleosis, these patients and their doctors might never consider the possibility that CFS was the cause of their symptoms.

The distinction between CFS and acute infectious mononucleosis is also crucial because, though a patient may not feel much of a difference between these two illnesses, they are quite different diseases. All too frequently, because a patient's blood test for acute infectious mononucleosis has, typically, come back negative, the patient's complaints are dismissed by a doctor who excludes the possibility of a chronic mononucleosis-*like* illness.

Nonetheless, I realize that the comparison of mononucleosis and CFS is inevitable, what with the symptoms, such as fatigue and malaise, being so similar. Even I still use the comparison at times when talking to a layperson, because it helps me to explain my unique and relatively unknown illness by likening it to one that is easier to recognize and understand.

CFS AND EPSTEIN-BARR

Many physicians used to believe that the principal infectious agent of CFS was the Epstein-Barr virus (EBV), and in fact, the syndrome was most frequently referred to as chronic Epstein-Barr virus (CEBV). Today, however, most researchers no longer believe that the EB virus is the sole causative agent, though it is still too early to totally negate the roll of EBV in this syndrome.

The reasons EBV is no longer considered the main culprit are many, but two stand out. First, patients with this syndrome are just as likely to test positive for other conditions, such as cytomegalovirus, herpes simplex, or measles.

The second reason is that researchers no longer see a correlation between a positive blood test for EBV and the presence of CFS symptoms. The Epstein-Barr virus was originally thought to cause CFS because it was believed that most patients with CFS tested positive for the virus. It is now known, however, that normal, healthy individuals can have similar blood results to those of CFS patients, and that there are CFS patients whose blood tests reveal they have never even had EBV.

There *is* a true form of chronic Epstein-Barr virus, but it differs from CFS. It is a rare and severe illness with major organ involvement, and is typically accompanied by more serious conditions such as chronic hepatitis, pneumonia, anemia, and sometimes lymphoma. These patients have test results that demonstrate an exceedingly high presence of active EBV infection, much higher than in CFS patients.

Dr. Straus of the NIH considers it possible that some CFS patients may be found to have a milder form of this chronic Epstein-Barr infection—especially those patients who lack certain antibodies (such as EBNA) to the EB virus, or those whose illness started as acute mononucleosis. The typical CFS patient, however, does not lack these antibodies, and the onset of CFS is usually correlated with illnesses other than mononucleosis, such as the flu or bronchitis. In others, symptoms developed more gradually, without an obvious link to any disease. The majority of CFS patients are not believed to suffer from a chronic EB virus infection.

Therefore, while many doctors still believe that the EB virus may be involved in some way, it is no longer thought to be the driving force behind CFS. If it does play a role, it is probably not a primary one. There may be other viruses involved, or CFS may be caused by some sort of immune dysfunction.

CFS—CONTAGIOUS OR NOT?

While the exact cause of CFS is still unknown, the good news is that it does not appear to be contagious. Since both Shawn and I have CFS, it may seem odd for me to claim that we are no more infectious than the average person. But studies have shown that transmission of chronic fatigue syndrome between family members is unusual. To date, we know of only a few other married couples with CFS. The vast majority of spouses, siblings, relatives, or friends of CFS patients don't become ill. Shawn and I may have become infected from a common source. And even though the odds were against it, our doctors think we probably both have immune incompetence toward this syndrome, or that we both happen to have a genetic predisposition to become ill with CFS.

VIRUSES AND THE IMMUNE SYSTEM

Even though the cause of CFS remains a mystery, most of the theories center around viral or immunologic origin. Therefore, before I deal with some of the possible causes of this syndrome, it will help to give you some information about viruses in general, as well as an overview of the human immune system.

Viruses are small organisms, about one ten-thousandth the size of a pinhead, and are visible only through a powerful electron microscope. They are biologically simple organisms, consisting of an outer protein coat surrounding inner genetic material. Despite their simplicity, there is still much that is unknown about viruses and viral infections.

Patients, accustomed to being treated for bacterial infections with simple and effective medicines, such as penicillin, always seem surprised to learn how little modern medicine can do to treat viral infections. While bacterial infections invade the organs of the body, viruses invade the actual cells. They invade the cells because, unlike bacteria, they are unable to reproduce on their own. They need to genetically hijack the reproductive capability of body cells in order to propagate. Since viruses live within the cells of the body, however, drugs that are able to destroy a virus may also destroy the cells that contain that virus.

Viruses infect the body in many different ways. Some are airborne; infection results from beathing air that contains the virus. Others, such as HIV, the virus associated with AIDS, are transmitted through the blood or by sexual contact. The EB virus is typically spread through saliva; hence the nickname for mononucleosis is "the kissing disease of amorous adolescents." (The EB virus can also be spread through blood transfusions and possibly through other forms of intimate contact; this is not known for sure.)

Each type of virus has an affinity for a particular cell in the body. It is usually a cell that is biochemically susceptible to invasion by that virus. The EB virus attacks the B cells, one type of white blood cell that is part of the immune system. This disrupts the normal immune response.

After a virus invades the body, it touches down on a cell much the same way a mosquito lands on your arm. It then enters that cell either by being absorbed directly across the cell membrane—the outer "skin" of the cell, as it were—or by puncturing the cell like a mosquito. Next, it releases its own genetic material into the cell.

Once inside, the virus quickly and effectively goes about the task of transforming an otherwise normal and healthy cell into a miniature virus factory. It reprograms the reproductive machinery of the cell to manufacture thousands of new viruses. What happens next depends on the type of virus as well as the type of cell infected. Some types of viruses, called lytic viruses, cause the host cell to burst open and die, unleashing a new generation of viruses to continue the struggle of invade and conquer.

Other viruses can cause a latent infection. (This is what typically occurs in mononucleosis.) These viruses are capable of immortalizing the host cell. In other words, the host cell still lives and reproduces, but with the virus inside it. The genetic material of the virus remains stably present inside the cell nucleus. When the cell divides, producing a new daughter cell, the virus also divides, becoming part of every new daughter cell. This allows the virus to reproduce itself perpetually, as long as the host cell lives. These viruses can create lifelong infections because, once inside the host cell, they can hide from detection by the immune system. Other types of viruses leave themselves vulnerable by bursting and destroying the very host cell they need in order to survive.

Still other viruses can cause infections that persist and reactivate. (Some doctors believe that this is the type of infection involved in CFS.) The host cell is still preserved intact as in latent infection; however, the virus is actively reproducing itself. New viral particles are released into the body, causing an increased and continuous immune response.

THE IMMUNE SYSTEM RESPONDS

Within hours after a virus enters the body, the immune system mobilizes for action. An incredibly complex sequence of separate yet interdependent events is set in motion, culminating in the destruction of the invading virus. While the immune system is still a perplexing and largely unexplored entity, enough is known to give us remarkable insight into the body's amazing ability to protect itself against infection.

The immune system has two basic functions: to recognize anything that may be detrimental to your health, and to respond protectively. This clever system not only protects against infections, but is able to distinguish between self and nonself—between what is you and what is not you—preventing the body's own cells from coming under attack by the immune system.

The immune system is able to recognize and respond to millions of different foreign intruders, referred to as antigens (an antigen being anything that triggers an immune response). The chief components of that response are called white blood cells. There are trillions of white blood cells in the body at any one time. The majority of them are stored in such areas as the spleen and lymph nodes, waiting to be called upon when needed. The relatively few that are circulating throughout the body act as sentinels, constantly on guard against anything that might do harm. There are many different classes of white blood cells. The most notable of these are divided into three groups, depending on the particular function they serve. These are the T cells, B cells, and the macrophages.

The T Cell

When a virus invades the body it is the circulating T cells that recognize it as a foreign antigen. The surface of every infecting antigen is different from anything else found in the body. When a T cell comes into contact with this antigen, it calls for reinforcements by releasing chemical signals into the blood-stream. (These messages can also be released by other cells, such as macrophages.) Some of these chemical signals, called lymphokines (also called cytokines), have been isolated and identified, and may sound familiar. These include interferon and interleukin I and II. These chemical messages have many known and unknown functions. They regulate and communicate with cells of the immune system. They warn the body that there is an infection present, alerting the stored white blood cells that their help is needed. They also warn the cells in the infected area about the presence of the virus, causing the cells to become resistant to penetration by the virus. Lymphokines inhibit the reproducing capability of those cells, thereby inhibiting the reproductive capability of any virus that has managed to enter a cell. Conversely, lymphokines are also capable of stimulating the reproductive capability of cells of the immune system at the same time they are impairing the reproductive capability of viruses. They also initiate the inflammatory response, which is familiar to anyone who has ever cut a finger.

When the skin of a finger is cut, the body becomes vulnerable to the invasion of millions of bacteria and viruses. In order to prevent this infection from spreading, lymphokines, as well as a chemical named histamine, are released. These chemicals increase blood flow to the infected area by dilating the blood vessels, speeding up the deployment of the stored white blood cells. While blood flow is increased, the infected area is simultaneously sealed off from the rest of the body, thereby containing the infection and preventing it from spreading. The increase of blood flow, with the subsequent closing off of the infected area, causes the finger to become red and swollen.

Typically, any infection associated with a cut finger is mild enough to be contained within hours, and the damaged area heals within days. However, many infections are not so easily contained. If the infection is severe enough, it may actually make you ill. There is usually a lag time of approximately two days before the body has marshaled the full strength of the immune system to destroy the invaders. During that time, the virus has the upper hand, making you sick by destroying healthy and vital cells. The virus also acts like a parasite, siphoning the food and energy so desperately needed by the cells of the body.

Viral infections cause many symptoms, one of which is fever. Fever serves many purposes, but one of its main functions is suspected to be fighting the infection. Many viruses are unable to function effectively at higher temperatures. The elevation of body temperature, therefore, aids in the battle against infection.

Another common result of viral infections is loss of appetite. One possible reason for this is that blood flow is rerouted from low-priority areas, such as the stomach, to high-priority areas that contain the virus. This allows speedy deployment of white blood cells. This decrease in blood flow to the stomach may be experienced as a decrease in appetite.

The worst symptoms of viral infections, especially with CFS, are the feelings of sickness and fatigue. There are many theories concerning the cause of these symptoms. They may be caused by the release of certain lymphokines, which are known to produce many symptoms similar to CFS. The feelings of sickness and fatigue may be the result of the abnormal functioning of the immune system. Another theory is that these feelings may be caused by the effect of viruses on specific cell components. (Many researchers in Britain are concentrating their efforts on the effect of CFS on the mitochondria of the cell. The mitochondria act as the powerhouse of the cell to supply its energy.) Another theory focuses on the incredible amount of energy being used to fight this microscopic war. The size of the combatants may be small, but the drain of your strength and the strain on your body are not. The typical weapons used in this war are cellular toxins and poisons, called cytotoxins. These toxins are used by the immune system to kill viruses and bacteria, but, because of their potency, they can also make you tired and ill.

T cells have more functions than merely the recognition of antigens. They also serve as a type of on/off switch for the immune system. Certain T cells, referred to as helper T cells, stimulate the immune system to fight infection. Other T cells, referred to as suppressor T cells, switch off the immune system once the infection is under control. Certain T cells also have the capability of fighting infections directly. These specialized cells, called cytotoxic T cells, have the ability to destroy viruses directly by releasing cytotoxins. Another class of T cells, referred to as natural killer cells, are also able to attack a virus immediately and form the first line of defense against foreign invaders.

The B Cell

B cells, another type of blood cell of the immune system, are also required to fight infection and, as with T cells, have many different functions.

The main function of B cells is to produce deadly proteins called antibodies. Antibodies are shaped like a Y and have very specific receptor sites on their surface, allowing them to recognize and attack one particular virus.

These antibodies fit into one particular virus the way a key fits into one particular lock. If the key is not engineered for that lock, it will not work. This specificity serves two purposes. It ensures that these powerful antibodies will attack only foreign antigens and not the cells of the body. It also serves as a type of memory system, allowing the immune system to remember a specific infectious agent. When the infection is over, the immune system retains these specific antibodies. If that particular strain of virus should ever invade the body again, the immune system will be able to respond quickly and powerfully, preventing a recurrence of that illness.

The ability of the immune system to remember and recognize past infections is the reason vaccinations against certain diseases are effective. For example, when an injection of a severely weakened or dead form of the polio virus is given, the dead virus is not able to cause the disease, but the body still produces antibodies that remain in the system. In the future, should the body become infected with the live polio virus, the immune system will respond quickly to destroy the virus, preventing contraction of the actual disease.

To date, five classes of antibodies have been identified. These antibodies, also referred to as immunoglobulins, each serve a different function. Immunoglobulin M, known as IgM, is the largest of the antibodies. It is also the first antibody produced during an infection. After a few days, the smaller, faster, and more mobile antibody known as IgG takes over. IgG is by far the most numerous of all the antibodies, comprising over 70 percent of the antibody total. IgA is an antibody most frequently found in the nose and mouth. It serves as the first line of defense against airborne infections. IgE is the antibody implicated in allergic reactions, and little is known about the IgD antibody.

Unlike T cells, B cells do not have the capability of attacking a virus directly. However, B cells produce a certain class of antibodies called neutralizing antibodies that can. B cells also produce another class of antibodies that, when combined with nine specialized proteins, called complement proteins, can achieve this same effect. These proteins, which circulate throughout the blood, are lethal toxins that do not have the safeguard of specificity that antibodies do. They destroy any cell they come in contact with. A fail-safe system is necessary in order to safely handle these deadly proteins; B cells are that fail-safe system.

These nine complement proteins, when taken individually, are safe and harmless in the same way that charcoal, potassium nitrate, and sulfur are safe and harmless; it's only when mixed together that they become gunpowder. B cells are responsible for combining these proteins into a lethal concoction and holding that concoction to the virus to be destroyed.

Other classes of antibodies that are summoned to the infected area as reinforcements serve to incapacitate the virus, preventing it from entering the body's cells. They also attach themselves to the virus and serve as a recognition flag, or signal, enabling other, more lethal cells of the immune system to easily recognize and destroy the virus.

As I have mentioned, B cells produce specific antibodies that destroy specific viruses. But one B cell would not be able to produce enough antibodies to handle thousands of viruses. It needs help. This help comes from a third type of white blood cell, called macrophages, which are discussed in more detail below.

Macrophages release a chemical called transfer factor. This is a message telling other B cells to employ the same specific killing capability as the first B cell. In other words, transfer factor stimulates other B cells to become identical clones of the first B cell. It "transfers" the genetic capability to fight a specific virus from one cell to another.

Macrophages

Macrophages, the largest of the white blood cells, have many functions. One of the most important is phagocytosis. This means that these cells can destroy viruses by swallowing and engulfing them whole, kind of like an immunologic Pac-Man.

These scavengers are indispensable to the immune system because they not only engulf viruses, they engulf all the debris that has collected in the infected area. For, as in any war, the dead and debris of battle are strewn everywhere. There are poisons and toxins, as well as bits and pieces of the winners and the losers. If this decaying debris were not removed, the area would be no better than a toxic waste dump, poisoned and inhospitable to life. Macrophages remove all this toxic matter from the site of the infection, allowing it to heal and be restored.

SOME POSSIBLE CAUSES OF CFS

Even though a chronic mononucleosis-like illness has been described in the medical literature for decades, for all intents and purposes CFS is a new discovery. At this point in our knowledge, there are far more questions than answers to the perplexing problem of understanding CFS. Mostly what we have is speculation. For that reason, it is important to remember that what this next section describes are theories, not concrete facts.

A Role for Epstein-Barr?

Though the Epstein-Barr virus is no longer considered to be the sole causative agent of CFS, many doctors believe it does play a role in some way. I feel it is therefore useful to include some information about this virus.

Epstein-Barr virus is named for two of the English scientists who first isolated it. It is very common and thought to be responsible for a wide range of diseases found throughout the entire world—diseases ranging in severity from the deadly to the benign.

The most severe illnesses EBV has been linked to are two cancers: Burkitt's lymphoma (a lymph node cancer found mainly in Africa) and nasopharyngeal carcinoma (a nose and throat cancer found mainly in Asia). It is important to note that the vast majority of Americans infected by the EB virus do not develop cancers. These two cancers strike very specific population groups that have a genetic predisposition to them. The odds are remote that anyone with CFS would develop cancer caused by the EB virus.

In contrast to these serious manifestations is the more typically benign infection, mononucleosis. In fact, many people have such mild and transient infections that their illness resolves practically unnoticed.

At one time or another, most everyone is exposed to the EB virus. In fact, infection with this virus is so common that 90 percent of the adult population of the United States over age thirty has been infected. And yet, the EB virus is not as easy to catch as it sounds. Most doctors believe that a casual kiss or living in the same household with someone who is ill would not pass on the infection. It's just that with the EB virus so ubiquitous, 90 percent of us run into it eventually.

Typically, within the first few months of the initial infection, most patients are shedding the EB virus. Shedding means that the virus is active and being excreted in the saliva, which may increase the likelihood of that individual transmitting the virus to another person. However, even healthy people can spread the virus. Many people who have recovered from an initial infection can have asymptomatic reactivation of the virus. This means that these people are shedding the virus intermittently, but do not experience any symptoms from the reactivation of that virus. In fact, a random sampling of the adult population will reveal that at any one time, approximately 20 percent are shedding the virus. In other words, you can become infected with the EB virus from a healthy person shedding the virus as well as from someone who has an obvious illness, such as mononucleosis.

Epstein-Barr virus is a member of the herpes family of viruses, which also includes herpes simplex 1 and 2 (the first causes oral herpes, creating cold sores; the second is responsible for the infamous genital herpes); varicella-zoster virus (which causes chicken pox and shingles); cytomegalovirus (known as CMV, which causes an illness similar to mononucleosis); and a relatively new herpesvirus called human herpesvirus 6 (or HHV6). It is not yet known for sure, but HHV6 may cause diseases similar to those caused by the Epstein-Barr virus.

I mention these viruses not only because they are distant relatives to EBV, but also because they have one very important characteristic in common. Once you have become infected with any type of herpesvirus, you remain infected for life. With all herpesviruses, the body typically develops immunity against further outbreaks of the disease associated with that virus. In other words, the virus is still present in the body, but in a latent and inactive form.

Despite that immunity, however, it can happen that the disease associated with a latent herpesvirus recurs. For example, some people continue to have outbreaks of oral or genital herpes. One suggested reason for this is that some people's immunity may not be adequate to prevent symptomatic recurrences. It is therefore theorized that patients with CFS may be experiencing a reactivation of an EBV infection due to some environmental stress or genetic susceptibility.

EBV may be one of *many* possible trigger mechanisms of CFS rather than the actual cause. Other trigger factors could be other viruses, such as HHV6, or even nonviral agents. In Britain, much of their investigation into the cause of this illness (known there as myalgic encephalomyelitis) has been focused on the Coxsackie virus. This virus usually enters the body through the mouth and multiplies in the stomach and the intestines. This virus is typically benign and self-limiting, and most often causes symptoms no worse than a common cold. However, this virus has been found to be the cause of Bornholm disease (also known as epidemic myalgia). This disease has many similar symptoms to CFS such as fatigue, mental confusion, fever, headache, and muscle pains, and this is why the Coxsackie virus is being viewed as a possible cause of CFS.

It is also possible that EBV may be a cofactor. In other words, there may be more than one virus involved, the two acting synergistically: both flourishing together where neither would flourish alone. Or, EBV infection may allow another virus to gain a foothold. If there *is* more than one virus involved, it is hoped that they can be isolated and treated with antiviral drugs.

Some doctors think that HHV6 may be a cofactor in CFS, or that it may be solely responsible. CFS patients may be fighting both HHV6 and another virus at once. There is evidence that suggests that HHV6 is more prevalent in CFS patients than in the general population. However, since the percentage of healthy people with HHV6 is substantial, the significance of this has not yet been determined.

The "New-Strain" Theory

Another theory holds that people with CFS are infected with a new and different strain of a known virus. It is believed that there is something genetically different about this strain that makes it particularly virulent and more difficult to destroy.

In fact, genetically different strains of viruses are not uncommon. This can be observed in the flu viruses. Typically, the body immunizes against recurring illness by the same virus, yet people are susceptible to the flu every year. This is because the influenza viruses are genetically different every year. The body builds immunity to one strain one year, but fails to recognize the new strain the next. I realize that this makes viruses seem almost intelligent, but they are no different from any other organism. In order to survive, they are constantly adapting to better suit their environment.

Therefore, CFS patients may, in fact, have encountered a different strain of virus than what is typically found. Whether this different strain is particularly stronger, or is just not easily recognized, it is overwhelming the immune system. Even if this theory were true, however, it still does not explain our inability to recover from this infection. With the flu virus, though the body may be unable to recognize each new strain immediately, in the end the immune system does prevail. Not so, it seems, with CFS.

The Hormonal Theory

It is believed that viruses can also disrupt the body's ability to regulate the production of hormones by the endocrine system. (The endocrine system is comprised of glands, like the adrenal glands, which among other things are responsible for metabolism—the conversion of food into energy.) There are endocrine pathways that produce hormones, like cortisol, which may be dysfunctioning. The body's reaction to cortisol has been implicated in depression and may indicate a similar dysfunction in CFS. There is ongoing research by the NIH into the effects of viral illnesses on hormone pathways.

Immune-Dysfunction Theories

Because so much is unknown regarding this syndrome, we must be wary of assuming that whenever a CFS patient demonstrates the presence of a virus like EBV or HHV6, the cause of the syndrome has been discovered. In fact, the presence of a virus may be more indicative of an immune abnormality. In other words, whatever is causing the syndrome may allow a usually dormant virus to reactivate. This may explain why patients with CFS have been shown to respond positively to tests for so many different viruses or diseases, such as EBV, CMV, herpes simplex, and measles.

One set of theories holds, therefore, that CFS patients have some sort of immune dysfunction. Some crucial link in the immunologic chain of events is defective, missing, or altered. From reading even my simplified overview of the immune system, you can see that it is a very complex system. There are literally hundreds of different ways the immune system might be defective. The body needs every part of the immune system to function cohesively and properly in order to control infection. Each individual part is vital to the whole. CFS patients may have too few or too many suppressor T cells. There may be deficient or absent IgG antibodies. The inflammatory control may be lost or T cell recognition may be blocked. Maybe the immune system was depressed when the infection was first contracted, and it hasn't been able to recover since.

There is evidence that does suggest immune abnormalities in CFS patients compared to healthy individuals. For example, some patients have deficiencies in one of the subclasses of IgG antibodies. Other patients exhibit a higher number of circulating immune complexes (an immune complex is the joining of an antibody to an antigen). Some patients have abnormal ratios of helper T cells to suppressor T cells. And still other patients exhibit suppressed activity of unique classes of cytotoxic white blood cells such as neutralizing antibodies and natural killer cells.

There is a theory that sustained activation of the immune system may cause CFS symptoms to persist, even though the original causative agent is no longer active. In other words, there may be some dysfunction that does not allow the immune system to relax. It is possible that, like a car engine that will not shut off, the immune system is overreacting, wearing us out, because it is not recognizing that the infection has been brought under control.

Perhaps the immune system is overproducing lymphokines, such as interferon or interleukin, or is producing them long after the initial infection has been resolved. These lymphokines are used to fight infection and regulate the immune system, and are thought to produce many of the symptoms associated with CFS, such as fatigue, feverishness, malaise, muscle aches, and depression.

It is interesting to note that lymphokines are not released during every type of infection. For example, they are not released during infection with German measles or the common cold, illnesses that do not share the flulike symptoms of CFS. And yet, in infections that are known to precede the onset of CFS, such as the flu or mononucleosis, lymphokines are produced.

There may also be a genetic defect in the immune system. People with CFS may have inherited an inability to fight this particular infection in the same way others inherit sickle-cell anemia or Down's syndrome. There may also be genetic signals that keep individual viruses dormant. If latent viruses are involved in causing CFS, there may be a defect in the molecular on/off switch that controls this infection.

The Allergy Theory

This immune-related theory suggests that patients with CFS may have an allergic hypersensitivity that has somehow become unmasked. As many as 80 percent of CFS patients do have a history of allergies, compared to 15 percent of the general population. When an allergic reaction occurs, the IgE antibody binds to the allergen (the foreign substance that induces the allergy), causing a release of histamine. Histamine is responsible for many of the symptoms related to allergy, such as fatigue, headaches, respiratory problems, and so on. Since such a high percentage of CFS patients have allergies, it may be possible that their immune systems are overreacting to the presence of general infectious agents in the same way they overreact to the presence of allergens.

Whatever the mechanism, the common thread in all these theories is that some part of the immune system is being either inhibited or overworked. It may even be too simple to suppose that the cause of CFS is that the immune system is either overactive or underactive. It is possible that CFS may be caused by a combination of the two. In fact, current data indicate that in some CFS patients, some immune functions are overactive while others are normal or underactive. The overall functioning of the immune system is still intact, which explains our ability to fight off other infections, but some vital immunologic response, critical to the control of whatever infection causes CFS, is missing.

As with viral theories, we must also exercise caution in regard to immune-related theories. After all, it is even difficult to know whether immune abnormalities are the cause of CFS or are a result of the disease process itself.

Psychological Involvement

There is still considerable debate going on regarding the role that neuropsychological factors play in CFS. There is information that prevents us from disregarding this possibility. Clearly there is a link between the psyche and the immune system. Patients who are depressed have been shown to be immunologically different from nondepressed patients. Therefore, depression may play an immunologic role in many of the symptoms of CFS. I am not arguing that depression isn't a natural consequence of severe and chronic illness or that depression can't affect us physically and immunoligically. However, I do not feel that depression is actually responsible for our chronic illness. Too many people feel that it is a cause rather than a result of this syndrome.

It is true that stress and depression can have a dramatic effect on the body's ability to recover from infection. It is equally true that there may indeed be a subset of patients whose symptoms can be linked to depression and psychological problems. There may be psychological components that contribute to many of the symptoms of this illness, and there may even be patients whose psychological profiles make them more susceptible to developing CFS. However, I do not feel that the majority of CFS patients can be explained away by categorizing them as simply depressive or psychoneurotic. This just is not consistent with the physical, immunologic, and historical findings.

With so many theories to choose from, who can predict which—if any—will turn out to be the cause of CFS? Perhaps several of these theories, as opposed to only one, may be correct. It is my opinion that researchers will one day discover that CFS is not really one specific illness, but rather a broad classification, encompassing many different subclasses. These subclasses will be similar symptomatically, but will probably have different causes. In other words, although CFS patients share the same symptoms, the reasons why they are sick will be found to be different.

While this theory is just my opinion, there are plenty of precedents for it. Diabetes, for example, is divided into more than one type. Diabetics have an insulin problem; they are not able to break down blood sugar, the basic energy source for the body. Some diabetics are unable to produce insulin in their pancreas and are treated with insulin injections. Others are able to produce the insulin, but are unable to utilize it. These people are usually treated with diet and exercise.

Similarly, we may all share a common syndrome referred to as CFS. We may have a common history and common symptoms as well. We may even share the same virus. But the reason that each of us is chronically ill may be completely different, and therefore different treatments would be required. Certain people may have immune deficiencies and may need a drug to bolster their immune system. Other people, who are experiencing chronic reactivation of one or more viruses, may need an antiviral drug.

There are countless theories for the cause of CFS. Right now, any or all of them may be right. It will be interesting to discover which, if any, most closely explains the cause of CFS.

4

Diagnosis

To the dismay of many doctors, chronic fatigue syndrome remains very much a "symptoms" disease. When making a diagnosis, doctors still must rely more on what a patient feels than on any objective evidence. There are no blood tests or other laboratory methods to determine who is suffering from CFS.

Unfortunately, many doctors, trained as scientists and therefore disinclined to believe what cannot be objectively verified, hesitate to rely exclusively on the subjective reports of their patients. In fact, this is one of the difficulties in obtaining research grants to study CFS. The powers that be are reluctant to finance research into an illness without an objective method of determining who has that illness. It is unfortunate that so much emphasis has been placed on the lack of a diagnostic blood test for CFS. Dr. Straus, of the NIH, points out that there are many precedents for the study of diseases for which there are no blood tests, such as psychiatric disorders and multiple sclerosis.

It has been my good fortune to be under the care of doctors who are not threatened by medical uncertainties. They remind

57

me of the old country doctors who knew that their patients were the best source of information when making a diagnosis.

It can be argued that the doctors who practiced fifty or sixty years ago had no other choice but to listen to the speculations of their patients. They did not have access to the amazing technology that today makes diagnosis an exact science. While this is certainly true, it also seems true that people have never been as dissatisfied with the quality of medical care as they are today.

Their dissatisfaction, it seems to me, stems from the fact that too few doctors are willing to listen to their patients. The old country doctors, usually responsible for their patients' total care, thoroughly knew each and every patient and were often called upon to dispense advice as much as medicine. But today, many doctors have forgotten how to treat the whole person. Modern medicine examines a patient and sees a hundred different specialties. There is a doctor for feet, one for knees, one for skin, and even one for the brain, but there isn't a doctor to care for the whole patient.

I don't mean to imply that the explosion of medical technology is not beneficial. We have gained many wonderful tools that help eliminate pain and suffering. But I am apprehensive when doctors rely on technology to the degree that the patient seems almost superfluous. I have seen too many people hurt when their illness was callously dismissed simply because a blood test could not determine what was causing their pain. I understand that doctors must consider all the possibilities when making a diagnosis—including hypochondria. But the tendency to doubt the existence of illnesses they are unable to understand or diagnose is painfully wrong. All I ask of doctors is that they be willing to admit the possibility that they don't know the cause of an illness rather than automatically disputing its legitimacy.

If you suspect that you have CFS, but have been unable to find a doctor who believes in this syndrome, continue searching until you find one who does. Your doctor should be someone you can depend on for help, advice, and support. When you do finally find a caring physician—and there are many wonderful ones out there—treat him with respect. Patients often vent their impatience and frustration on their doctors when medicine has little to offer in the way of treatments. Antagonism is not conducive to establishing a healthy working relationship.

ACHIEVING A DIAGNOSIS

Even though I've stated that symptoms are important in making a CFS diagnosis, I don't want any readers to decide they have CFS just because they feel sick and tired. Work with your doctor. The symptoms of CFS are general enough to be associated with a multitude of other illnesses—including many that require immediate attention.

The Major Criteria

In their March 1988 article in the *Annals of Internal Medicine*, "Chronic Fatigue Syndrome: A Working Case Definition" (see Appendix D), Dr. Gary Holmes and a group of leading researchers concluded that for a patient to fit the definition for CFS, two major criteria, as well as a number of minor criteria, have to be met. It's important to remember that this working definition was established in order to be sure that investigators study groups of patients who are comparable to those studied by other investigators. Therefore, while not intended to be strictly diagnostic, the criteria they have established are used to identify the typical CFS patient.

The first major criterion is that all other conditions that might produce similar symptoms must have been ruled out through physical examination, an evaluation of the patient's history, and appropriate labwork. The following are some of these other possible causes:

1. Chronic inflammatory disease (such as hepatitis)
2. Autoimmune disease (such as arthritis)
3. Neuromuscular disease (such as myasthenia gravis or multiple sclerosis)
4. Cancer (such as nasopharyngeal carcinoma, Burkitt's lymphoma, Hodgkin's disease, or other lymphomas)
5. AIDS
6. Fungal disease, bacterial disease (such as Lyme disease or tuberculosis), and parasitic disease (such as toxoplasmosis)
7. Endocrine disease (such as diabetes or hypothyroidism)
8. Localized infection
9. Chronic psychiatric disease (such as endogenous depression, schizophrenia, or chronic use of major tranquilizers or antidepressive medications)
10. Drug dependency or abuse
11. Side effects of a chronic medication or toxic agent (such as a pesticide or heavy metal)
12. Other known or defined chronic pulmonary (lung), cardiac (heart), gastrointestinal (stomach and intestinal), hepatic (liver), renal (kidney), or hematologic (blood) disease

I realize this is an intimidatingly long list of diseases. This is because the researchers who authored this paper wanted to ensure that patients are not misdiagnosed as having CFS, when in fact they might have some other affliction. Check with your physician to determine which of these diseases should concern you.

The second major criterion by which CFS is defined requires that there be a "new onset of persistent or relapsing, debilitating fatigue or easy fatigability in a person who has no previous history of similar symptoms," and that the fatigue not resolve with bed rest. This fatigue must have lasted at least six months and be severe enough to impair average activity by at least 50 percent.

The Minor Criteria

If the above criteria for persistent and extreme fatigue have been met, with tests such as general blood tests, urinalysis, and clinical evaluations being normal and unremarkable, and if other possible diseases have been ruled out, then the two major requirements of a working definition of CFS have been satisfied. But there are also the following minor criteria to be met:

1. Mild fever with oral temperature readings between 99.5 and 101 degrees Fahrenheit. Higher temperature readings are not considered compatible with CFS and should prompt studies for other causes of illness.
2. Sore throat
3. Painful lymph nodes in the neck or armpits. Lymph nodes greater than two centimeters in diameter are not compatible with CFS and suggest other causes.
4. Unexplained generalized muscle weakness
5. Muscular discomfort and pain
6. Prolonged (longer than twenty-four hours) generalized fatigue following levels of exercise that would have been easily tolerated by the patient before becoming ill
7. Generalized headaches, different from those experienced before the onset of illness
8. Migratory joint pain without joint swelling or redness
9. Neuropsychological complaints such as inability to concentrate, confusion, difficulty thinking, depression, irritability, forgetfulness, intolerance of light, and transient, partial visual blindness
10. Sleep disturbance, either too much or too little
11. The patient describing the onset of symptoms as having developed rapidly, over a few hours or a few days.

A patient need not have all of these minor requirements in order to fit the working definition of CFS; eight or more of the eleven will do. If eight or more are not present, the definition can still be satisfied if the patient reports at least six and a doctor can document two of the three following physical criteria: low-grade fever, sore throat, and palpable or tender lymph nodes.

Remember that this definition of CFS was established to provide guidelines for the study of this syndrome. Even if you do not meet some of the requirements, the intention was not to exclude you from a diagnosis. Although you would not fit the case definition for purposes of research, that does not necessarily mean that you do not have CFS. If you have ruled out other causes and have extreme fatigue, as well as some of the other accompanying symptoms, then there is a chance you have CFS. Until more is known about this affliction, and accurate diagnostic tests are developed, there will never be a foolproof method of determining who does and does not have this affliction.

THE MONOSPOT TEST

Those patients with CFS who can relate their illness to mononucleosis typically tell their doctors that they have mononucleosis that never went away; they know of no other way to describe it. Most of these patients are given the standard monospot blood test for mononucleosis. Unfortunately, this test does not diagnose CFS.

CFS is a completely different illness from mononucleosis, and too many doctors, unaware of this fact, wrongly assume that a negative result on the monospot test rules out the possibility of a chronic mononucleosis-like illness. As my own experience demonstrates, that is not necessarily the case.

THE EBV SEROLOGY TEST

There is a blood test that doctors have used in the past for the diagnosis of CFS, called the EBV serology blood test. It measures the presence of *antibodies* to the Epstein-Barr virus, from which the presence of the actual virus can be inferred. However, most physicians no longer believe that this blood test is useful in diagnosing CFS. There are several reasons for this conclusion. Not all patients who *do* have CFS have abnormal test results, and there seems to be no correlation between test results and the presence of symptoms. In addition, many *healthy* individuals have abnormal EBV test results, and many CFS patients also have positive results to tests for other diseases, such as measles or cytomegalovirus. But while the EBV serology blood test may no longer be considered diagnostic for CFS, since most patients with this syndrome have had this test performed, and because many doctors still believe that the EB virus is involved in this syndrome in some way, a brief discussion of the test will help you understand its aims and interpret its results.

As the name EBV serology titer test suggests, this test detects the presence of antibodies specific for the EB virus and thus infers the presence of the virus. Since each antibody is uniquely engineered for one specific virus, doctors can tell if you have had EBV by determining if you have the specific antibodies for EBV. Titers are a measurement of the amount of antibodies present, given as a ratio, the second number doubling each time antibodies are detected (e.g. 1:10, 1:20, 1:40, 1:80, 1:160, 1:320, etc.). The higher the second number, the greater the amount of antibodies present. The test results will look something like this:

Remark — — — EB Virus

IgG to VCA	— 1:320
IgG to EA	— 1:40
IgG to EBNA	— 1:40

IgG to VCA stands for Immunoglobulin G to Viral Capsid Antigen (the capsid is the outer protective coat of the virus). Once infected, this titer will remain elevated for life. Usually this titer measures around 1:640 during the acute period and drops to somewhere around 1:160 within months to a few years. Healthy adults typically have VCA titers less than or equal to 1:160, but many patients with CFS have titers greater than 1:160.

IgG to EA stands for Immunoglobulin G to Early Antigen. This antigen appears early in an EBV infection. High levels of this temporary and transient antibody typically suggest recent infection. Early antigen is normally present only during acute Epstein-Barr virus infection and usually regresses to titers of less than 1:10 within two years.

IgG to EBNA stands for Immunoglobulin G to Epstein-Barr Nuclear Antigen. This antibody usually appears late in the infectious process and is normally indicative of a past infection. After a while, this antibody should remain at fairly high levels, somewhere around 1:40. Only a small percentage of CFS patients, such as myself, are classified as EBNA negative. This means that there are low or absent levels of EBNA, indicating an abnormal immune response because most people develop this antibody within a year after their initial infection.

In some CFS patients, titer abnormalities, while not diagnostically significant, can be useful. They can, for example, indicate a possible reactivation of the Epstein-Barr virus, or an abnormal immune response. The EBV serology test, then, can be helpful, but not in making a diagnosis.

Until sensitive and accurate diagnostic tests are developed, diagnosis of CFS will remain difficult. Please remember that I am not a doctor and only a doctor can make or exclude a diagnosis of CFS. So find a doctor you can trust, educate each other, and work closely together.

If you have been diagnosed with CFS, don't neglect to see your physician regularly and to routinely have complete blood work done. It is important to check periodically for the presence of other infections (such as AIDS, hepatitis, and others) and to monitor the state of your immune system. Even though blood tests are not yet able to determine how well your immune system is functioning, they can determine the overall state of the system. This is important because not every ache or pain should be attributed to CFS. You deserve to be followed closely by a physician so he can differentiate what is caused by CFS and what may be caused by some other condition.

5

Treatments

A waiting game! This illness has turned my life into a waiting game. Rather than revel in the joy of a healthy and happy life, I am forced to sit idly by with subdued anticipation in the hope that someone, somehow, somewhere will discover a cure for chronic fatigue syndrome.

When I first became ill, there were dozens of promising therapies just waiting to be tried. I took suggestions from most any source—from my doctor to my next-door neighbor. I tried everything, from aloe juice to Zovirax, confident that at least one of them would make me well. But as the years went by, I slowly exhausted the list and still have not found a cure for my illness.

I know that just over the horizon there are always promising new drugs. If they are safe, I am willing to try them. As of now, however, I know of nothing that can be considered the cure for CFS.

Now, this is not to say that people with CFS don't get well. On the contrary, I know of quite a few who have. Some recovered spontaneously, while others attribute their restored health to some of the treatments discussed in this chapter. Others using these treatments have achieved partial relief. If my experience is typical, however, to date nothing can be heralded as a surefire cure for CFS.

That there is no cure may come as a shock to some of you. I remember being told that I would just have to learn to live with my illness. I had no intention of learning to live with it! I was sure it was only a matter of time until I found a cure. When reality finally did sink in, so did depression and despair: My disease was incurable.

I know I have painted a gloomy picture, and you may feel as if all hope is lost. But take heart; our plight is not being ignored. The growing public awareness of our illness is sparking an increase in research funding. Many fine doctors throughout the country are striving to understand our disease. But finding effective treatments is time-consuming. Doctors are understandably reluctant to simply pump into their patients any new drug that comes along. Not only would this be unethical, it could also be dangerous to experiment haphazardly with potent and powerful drugs.

We are fortunate to be living in an age of unprecedented growth in medical knowledge. Not a day goes by without some increase in man's ability to heal his fellow man. We will benefit immensely from these advances even if they are not directed specifically toward our illness. The increased attention focused on viruses, from herpes to AIDS, can only help further our cause; as scientists unravel the secrets surrounding viruses, they may also unravel the secrets surrounding CFS. So don't be discouraged! I truly believe that in the not-too-distant future, safe and effective medications will be found.

As discussed in the chapter "Understanding Your Illness," the causes of CFS may differ from person to person. Therefore, the efficacy of a particular treatment should never be dismissed simply because it did not help someone else. As long as the treatment is safe, has a fairly good chance of making you better, and is approved by a competent physician, it is worth a try. Evaluate each and every potential therapy objectively; decide with your head, not with your heart. And be wary of anyone who seems more interested in your money than in your health: I have spent thousands of dollars chasing after worthless treatments because I was desperate to try anything to get well.

More than likely, you are already trying different treatments or may do so in the near future. I have a recommendation: familiarize yourself with the *Physician's Desk Reference (PDR)*. It is an important reference book used by doctors to obtain information about drugs. It lists recommended dosages, possible side effects, and contraindications (circumstances when you should not use that drug). The *PDR* can help you make informed decisions regarding drugs you might try. Your local library or your physician should have one. Don't be intimidated by the long lists of side effects; the *PDR* is required to list them all, no matter how unlikely or rare. Discuss them with your doctor to determine which side effects should concern you.

The one drawback of the *PDR* is that it is assembled by the pharmaceutical companies, not by outside experts in the field. Because of this, discuss any potential medication with your pharmacist and your physician. They are often the best sources of information about the dangers and benefits of a drug.

You may also want to contact the pharmaceutical company that makes the drug you are considering. Either a pharmacist or the *Physician's Desk Reference* can tell you which drug company makes a particular drug. Shawn and I did this with a number of the drugs we tried because we wanted to learn all we could about them. The pharmaceutical companies should be aware of possible risks as well as the proper use of their drugs. They are also aware of current research into the efficacy of their drugs in treating various illnesses. When we inquired, they were very helpful and were willing to answer any questions we had. Between your doctor, the *PDR*, a pharmacist, and the drug companies, you should be able to make wise decisions regarding any possible treatments.

Unlike in the chapter on symptoms, the therapies discussed below are not presented in any particular order—neither by their prevalence nor their efficacy. Since I am still ill, I have no preference for one over another.

GAMMA GLOBULIN

There are trials currently being conducted to determine the efficacy of gamma globulin in treating CFS. While the jury is still out, some people not only claim to feel better while they are on this treatment, but have regained their health as well.

As therapies go, gamma globulin has very few side effects and is not toxic to the body. However, the long-term use of very high dosages of any medicine should never be undertaken lightly; too little is known about the long-term effect of any medicine.

Gamma globulin is a concentration of some of the antibodies found in the blood. The name *gamma globulin* is another name for immunoglobulin, or antibodies. It is a blood product that is prepared by distilling, concentrating, and purifying the antibodies from the blood plasma (a part of the blood that doesn't contain any cells) of many different donors. It has a very high concentration of immunoglobulin G, known also as IgG, and lesser concentrations of other antibodies.

Specific antibodies are necessary to destroy specific viruses. If the body is deficient in some of these antibodies, it may be unable to control this infection. Gamma globulin is given in the hope that it will replace whatever antibodies may be deficient. In this way, the antibodies are transferred from one person to another, passing immunity from one to another.

This treatment may be especially beneficial for CFS patients who exhibit a deficiency in neutralizing antibodies of one or more of the subclasses of IgG antibodies. IgG can be divided into four subclasses, and some patients with CFS exhibit a deficiency in one of these four subclasses. Doctors are still not certain how much significance to place on subclass deficiency since the overall IgG levels are usually normal. But since gamma globulin does contain neutralizing antibodies as well as all four subclasses of IgG, in theory, this treatment could help.

Gamma globulin can be given either intravenously (IV) or by injection. Intravenous treatment is usually the preferred method because it delivers a greater amount of the medicine than does injection. If you receive this medicine intravenously, be prepared to spend quite a few hours at the hospital. There is a lot of medicine to be given, and it should be administered slowly to avoid any side effects. With any infusion, there is always a possibility of experiencing an adverse reaction. The rapid infusion of gamma globulin may induce an inflammatory or allergic response, such as fever, headache, chills, and nausea. Even though serious reactions are unusual, patients should be carefully monitored during their treatments.

The dosage of gamma globulin is weight dependent; the more you weigh, the greater the amount of medicine. I started at a low dosage and continued to increase the dosage to the maximum allowed within safe limits. Your physician can inform you of all the specifics.

One drawback of gamma globulin is that it is very expensive. When my wife and I were receiving the highest doses, the annual cost of the treatment was over $25,000 for each of us. Fortunately, we were both covered by insurance, so we did not have to worry about the bills. But if you are not as fortunate, there are still a number of options available.

You can try to become part of a clinical trial of gamma globulin. When hospitals and pharmaceutical companies do research to determine the effectiveness of a treatment, they use patients for that research. One benefit to the patient is that the treatment is free. If you are unable to take part in a clinical trial, you should discuss your financial limitations with the hospital. Many hospitals make special arrangements for people who are in financial need. They frequently operate on a sliding scale;

you pay according to what you can afford. So don't assume this treatment isn't available to you because of its cost.

Gamma globulin may be very slow in taking effect. Some patients see an improvement in two or three months, but others not for over a year. But Shawn and I received this treatment for approximately one and a half years, to no avail. I do know people with CFS, however, who claim to have been helped dramatically by this treatment.

Before moving on to the next therapy, I think it is important that I discuss what seems to be on everybody's mind these days: AIDS. With the raging paranoia surrounding this deadly disease, people are understandably reticent to use anything that is derived from a blood product. I know I was. Of course no doctor can give you a blanket guarantee, but my doctors assured me that the chance of contracting AIDS from gamma globulin is virtually nonexistent.

Almost all of the AIDS cases that have resulted from contaminated blood have been from transfusions of whole blood. Gamma globulin is considered safe not only because blood donors are now well screened for AIDS, but because it uses just a small fraction of the blood, which is processed through many stages of filtering, distillation, and purification. There is very little chance that the virus associated with AIDS could still remain.

Gamma globulin has been used for decades in treating immunodeficient patients. As of this writing, my doctor knows of no reported AIDS cases being linked to the use of this treatment. But this is still a question that only you can resolve. You, and you alone, have to weigh even the remote possibility of risk against the possible benefits.

ACYCLOVIR (ZOVIRAX)

Acyclovir is one of the new generation of safe and effective antiviral drugs available today. The effectiveness of this drug on many different viral infections is presently being tested. The National Institutes of Health (NIH) has researched its effect on CFS. Its use is predicated on the assumption that CFS is caused by the Epstein-Barr virus.

By calling this medicine an antiviral drug, I don't mean it will eliminate the virus from your body. If it is the EB virus that is causing CFS, the virus is with us for life. In lab tests, however, this drug has been able to prevent the Epstein-Barr virus from replicating. This would be especially effective if the cause of CFS is an inability to control the EB virus raging within the body. By preventing the virus from reproducing, this drug would give the immune system a chance to revitalize itself and gain the upper hand in this microscopic battle.

Both Shawn and I have received IV and oral acyclovir. I received it as part of a double-blind study conducted by the NIH. A double-blind study is a scientifically controlled study to ascertain objectively the efficacy of a drug. It is called "double-blind" because neither the patient nor the doctor knows when the drug is being given and when the placebo is given (a placebo is nothing more than a sugar pill and has no medicinal value). Administering drugs and placebos at different times or to different patients allows doctors to discover whether patients are feeling better simply because they believe the medicine can cure them, or because of the effect of the medicine itself. If the majority of patients feel better on the medicine and not the placebo, doctors can be sure that the medicine does, in fact, work.

The placebo effect is a very interesting phenomenon; the mind is tricked into healing the body. Some people in my study experienced the placebo effect. At first, I was terribly disappointed to learn that people with my illness tricked themselves into feeling better. I couldn't help thinking that if patients got well on nothing more than a sugar pill, fuel would be added to the fire of disbelief. It is bad enough that so many people think CFS is all in our minds, without giving them the proof to back up their claim. Then I realized that I was looking at this phenomenon the wrong way. Instead of regarding the placebo effect as a threat to the authenticity of my illness, I began to look at it as a wonderful testament to the power of hope and belief.

The brain is a marvelous organ, an unexplored treasure trove of healing riches. The innate intelligence to make us feel better is within our own bodies. We actually have the power to affect our own health. I am not suggesting that, like Peter Pan, we merely need to think happy thoughts. But the placebo effect does prove that we can have a positive impact on the way we feel.

I received intravenous acyclovir in the hospital, three times a day for seven days. The intravenous form of the drug is very powerful and gives this medicine the best possible chance of working. Immediately following this intravenous treatment, I took the less potent oral form of the drug for four weeks. Unfortunately, I did not feel better on either trial. In fact, the only way I could tell the difference between the drug and the placebo was that I felt worse on the drug. There are patients, however, who do claim to feel better on this medicine.

If you do feel better on acyclovir, you would have to continue with this treatment until a more permanent cure is found. If you stop taking the medicine, there is nothing to prevent the EB virus from replicating again. At present, Dr. Straus of the NIH cannot recommend acyclovir because he did not find it effective in his placebo-controlled trials. He could not encourage people to stay on this medication just because they think they feel better on it. The long-term use of this drug should be discussed with your doctor. One side effect to be especially aware of is the tendency for acyclovir to affect the kidneys. Kidney function should be monitored during treatment with this medication.

TRANSFER FACTOR

Transfer factor is a treatment that neither my wife nor I have tried, but would consider in the future. As of now, I do not have firsthand experience with this treatment.

Transfer factor is considered safe as far as side effects are concerned. It has been used for quite a few years, and most of its possible side effects are known. It is a blood product, however, and therefore there is a concern about AIDS. Transfer factor is not considered as safe as gamma globulin because it does not go through as many stages of purification as gamma globulin does, so even greater caution is necessary. Donors should be well screened for both hepatitis and AIDS.

Transfer factor is derived from the immune system, but they are not antibodies. It is believed to be a lymphokine product that is secreted by white blood cells to help fight infection. If CFS is caused by an inability to fight infection, this treatment may enable the immune system to learn this ability. It is hoped that it transfers the ability to fight this infection from someone who has successfully recovered from the illness to someone who has not.

If patients with CFS are missing some vital genetic or chemical piece of information, preventing the immune system from recognizing or controlling this particular infection, maybe that missing piece can be supplied by the transfer factor. In a sense, transfer factor teaches the immune system what to do. It causes the unsensitized white blood cells to become sensitized, and better qualified to deal with the virus. In other words, it transforms general lymphocytes into lethal ones.

This drug is injected intramuscularly, and it may take several injections before it takes effect. Once it does, the injections should not need to be continued as often. Once the immune system has been sensitized, it can recall this information. However, infrequent follow-up treatments will probably be necessary to maintain your health. As of this writing, I have heard only sketchy accounts of people with CFS experiencing some improvement with transfer factor.

CORTISONE

This is a drug that many people are familiar with. It is a commonly prescribed anti-inflammatory drug, often used in treating arthritis. It relieves the pain and swelling typically associated with the inflammatory response.

If, like arthritis, CFS is an autoimmune disease, cortisone may relieve some of its symptoms. For if it is an autoimmune disease, the real culprit of CFS is a defective immune system turning and attacking the body. While cortisone is not able to reverse an autoimmune disease, it can control and alleviate the symptoms.

Cortisone treatments would need to be continued if found effective, but the long-term use of cortisone should not be undertaken without careful consideration. It is a potent drug with many severe side effects. Prolonged use of high doses of this drug can cause bloating of the face and limbs, severe headaches, high blood pressure, muscle weakness, nausea, vomiting, and other side effects. While cortisone inhibits the inflammatory response, it also suppresses the immune system, leaving the body vulnerable to other infections.

I have taken cortisone two different times during the course of my illness. The first time I took it was about a year after I first became ill. I started at 40 milligrams the first week and decreased the dosage by 10 milligrams each week for four weeks. That's because the body, which usually produces its own cortisone, stops producing it when it detects an unusually high concentration of this drug. Cortisone is often administered in decreasing doses to allow the body the time needed to restart its own production.

Cortisone can create a feeling of euphoria, making it difficult to evaluate its effectiveness objectively. I felt a little better on the lower doses, but on the higher doses I experienced severe headaches, insomnia, and nausea.

Shawn, on the other hand, did seem to experience a permanent improvement with this treatment. It improved her health one whole step. She went from being deathly ill to being only horribly ill. If you have not had a severe case of CFS, this may not seem like much of a change, but in fact it was a major improvement.

The second time I took cortisone was about a year later. I was supposed to take 20 milligrams for one month, since I had experienced a slight improvement on the lower dosage. I had to stop the treatment during the second week, however, because the side effects, along with the symptoms of CFS, were just too much to bear.

VITAMINS

The therapeutic value of vitamins in treating illness has been hotly debated for years. I have heard soul-stirring testimonies chronicling the miraculous recuperative power of vitamins. And, in fact, I do believe some of these accounts. Linus Pauling, a noted scientist and Nobel laureate, swears to their efficacy, and Norman Cousins, a well-respected author, believes that they literally saved his life.

The basic need for vitamins is not in dispute. Everyone needs them in order to live. By definition, vitamins are essential nutrients that must be obtained externally; the body is not able to manufacture them on its own. What *is* disputed is whether or not enough of these essential vitamins can be obtained solely from the food we eat. Do we need to supplement our diet with vitamin pills?

This question, like most questions concerning the fundamental mysteries of life, is beyond my ability to answer. (I can't even figure out why I always get full eating broccoli but never eating ice cream!) It is unfortunate that doctors, whose opinions we value most, are often undereducated in the field of nutrition. It is equally unfortunate that the people who have the most training in nutrition may also have the greatest financial interest in pushing vitamins.

I suppose that if you have a vitamin deficiency or you're not eating nutritious meals, you may need supplemental vitamins. My mother and I went to a special clinic for vitamin therapy. We went through the full regimen of blood tests to determine which specific vitamins we were deficient in, as well as which ones might improve our health. We spent well over six hundred dollars and were taking up to forty vitamins a day. I stopped taking the vitamins after several months because they had no noticeable effect and were very expensive.

This does not mean that vitamins are a waste of time and money for everyone. But you should talk to your doctor before taking large doses of vitamins. Some, such as the A vitamins, can be toxic to your system when taken in large quantities.

I am not able to discuss the specific attributes of each and every vitamin. Hopefully, either your doctor or a nutritionist can help you with that. But I do think it is important to discuss the three supplements most frequently taken by people with CFS. They are L-lysine, vitamin C, and tryptophan.

L-lysine is purported to be effective in fighting herpes infections. I know of many people, myself included, who have tried it as a specific therapy for CFS. I am unaware of anyone who has experienced any improvement. Since it is not harmful, though, it may be worth a try.

Vitamin C is heralded as a cure for everything from colds to cancer. Norman Cousins has written a book documenting his miraculous cure from cancer by using megadoses of this vitamin. Shawn and I tried taking up to 25 grams a day of vitamin C, to no avail. There are patients, however, who do claim some benefit from the more powerful intravenous form of vitamin C.

While tryptophan is not touted as a cure, many individuals have found it to be helpful as a sleep aid. It is the amino acid that is found in milk. Since a warm glass of milk has been the home remedy for insomnia for generations, it stands to reason that tryptophan might be equally effective. Although I am not aware of any data on tryptophan, I have heard many people testify to its ability to induce sleep.

DIET

This is one area I am quite familiar with. There is hardly a diet claiming even the slightest therapeutic value that I haven't tried. The purpose of these diets is not weight loss, although this is usually claimed as an extra benefit. Rather, these diets are supposed to enable the body to function in a healthier manner.

Some of these diets claim to bolster the immune system. They hold that there are certain food groups, such as wheat, soy, and dairy products, that can cause allergic reactions. The immune system, which is the primary system involved in any type of allergic reaction, is weakened by these foods. You feel ill because your body is mistaking these foods as foreign invaders, attacking them as it would a virus. These strict diets eliminate the suspect foods, and also claim that other foods can actually bolster the immune system.

Another diet that is popular now is the yeast-free diet. Yeast, like bacteria, is normally found in the body and, in small quantities, poses no threat. However, if your immunity is low and yeast multiplies unchecked, a yeast infection could be triggered, making you ill. You put out the "fire" by eliminating the fuel. Anything containing yeast is completely restricted. I was amazed to learn how prevalent yeast is. It is found not only in bread, but in pasteurized milk, many vitamins, cheese, canned goods, alcohol, enriched pasta, many foods containing sugar, and a host of other food products.

Another popular diet claims that the improper combination of food groups actually robs the body of energy. You feel weak and tired because your digestive system works too hard to digest miscombined foods. On this diet, you are not supposed to combine certain food groups—namely, proteins, carbohydrates, or dairy products—in the same meal. For example, meat should not be eaten with potatoes, or bread with cheese.

There are many other health-conscious diets, such as vegetarian diets. Unfortunately, I have not found the cure for CFS to be as simple as changing my eating habits. My feeling about special diets is the same as any other treatment I might consider. As long as it is safe, it is worth a try.

While Shawn and I did not experience any improvement through these diets, it has to be healthier to eat cauliflower rather than candy. We try to combine the nutritionally sound information from all of these diets. We still love our ice cream, but we eat many more fruits and vegetables than we used to. Although diets may not cure CFS, proper nutrition is essential to enable the body to heal itself. And if you do unknowingly suffer from food allergies or yeast infections, these diets may, in fact, be very beneficial.

CLINICAL ECOLOGY

Clinical ecologists believe that the environment can literally make a person ill. The chemicals in tap water may be polluting your body. The food you eat may be causing allergic reactions and suppressing your immune system. Even the air you breathe may be filled with harmful chemicals. Nothing is free from suspicion. They believe that environmental stresses overload the immune system and increase susceptibility to disease.

Shawn and I went to a clinical ecologist in New York City. We underwent extensive testing to determine what we were allergic to as well as what toxic chemicals might be making us ill. Aside from suggesting changes of diet and environment, this clinical ecologist gave us nystatin, an antifungal drug, to control yeast infections. He also claimed to have had a lot of success using injections of flu vaccine, which he said encouraged the production of antibodies that relieve certain symptoms associated with CFS.

I was informed by this doctor that I was a highly allergic person, but when I had allergy testing done at the NIH, I was not found to be allergic to one single thing. I don't want to imply that clinical ecologists are frauds. I really do believe that the environment can make a person ill, and that taking steps to eliminate toxins, allergens, and poisons from one's environment can only be beneficial. However, Shawn and I spent a lot of money without receiving any noticeable benefit.

CHIROPRACTIC

I have been under chiropractic care for three years. I began this treatment in the hope that it would make me well. I no longer continue treatment for that reason; I continue because I feel better under chiropractic care. Chiropractors believe that there is an innate intelligence in the body. They do not seek to cure any specific illness, or even merely to relieve backaches as is commonly believed. Their purpose is to allow the entire body to function at its best.

The central control network of the body is the nervous system. Nerves connect every organ of the body to enable them to function together as one unit. When those nerves are pinched, they become like a hose with a kink in it, unable to let the water of life flow through. Nerves become pinched when the bones of the spine become twisted or misaligned. This is referred to as a vertebral subluxation. Chiropractors reset these bones into their normal positions, thereby removing the pressure on the nerves. When the nerves are free from any interference, every part of the body will be able to function in a healthier manner.

Whatever your feelings on the philosophy of chiropractic, it does boast some amazing results. There are examples of people finding relief from a wide-ranging scope of ailments. While Shawn and I are obviously not well, we have noticed some significant changes. Though they are unrelated to CFS, many of the aches and pains we used to put up with have disappeared.

ACUPUNCTURE

Acupuncture is similar to chiropractic in its belief in the body's innate intelligence to heal itself. Rather than manipulating the spine, however, acupuncturists insert very fine needles into strategic areas of the body. These areas are believed to be crucial points important to the balance, function, and energy of the body. Disease results from a blockage of these points, and health will only be restored when the balance of the body is restored.

There is some scientific evidence to support the claims of acupuncture. For example, the human body is able to produce natural painkillers and hormones that are vital to a state of health. It is believed that the insertion of these needles stimulates the release of these chemicals, thereby making you feel better.

Shawn and I are currently undergoing acupuncture treatments. While we have not yet seen any change in the symptoms of our illness, Shawn has received some relief from her asthma, and I have been helped with my digestive problems.

LYMPHOKINES

In Chapter 3, "Understanding Your Illness," I discussed the role of lymphokines in the immune system. The lymphokines I listed were interferon, and interleukin I and II. Researchers have not only isolated these chemicals, they have also been able to produce them in large enough quantities to test their effectiveness on many different diseases.

Since lymphokines are normally released by the immune system, these drugs would be used to bolster the effectiveness of the immune system. Even though lymphokines are a naturally occurring body product, when given artificially they are very potent drugs and have many severe side effects.

I am not considering trying these drugs at this time because there are still too many unknowns, especially in their application to CFS. Since these drugs are still experimental, I doubt that your doctor can prescribe them. I mention lymphokines only because I have heard that some of the more desperate CFS patients are considering them as a possible treatment, and also because you will probably be hearing about new and different applications of these drugs in the future.

TRICYCLIC ANTIDEPRESSANTS

Tricyclic antidepressants have been used for years by psychiatrists to help alleviate depression. In lower doses, these drugs may also relieve some of the neurological symptoms of CFS. I have tried two different antidepressants, called Pamelor and Sinequan, for a total of seven months. I did not experience any significant change in my symptoms.

However, I do know of a few people who are on tricyclic antidepressants and have experienced some improvement. In fact, Shawn feels that Pamelor is helping her. Her throat and glands are less swollen and painful, her energy level is slightly improved, and the malaise has lessened. It is not a cure, but it is offering some relief.

In low doses, short-term use of tricyclic antidepressants is considered safe, but they can have serious side effects (especially with long-term use) and need to be prescribed and followed by a physician experienced in their use. The only side effects I experienced were merely unpleasant: a dry mouth, weight gain, and mild insomnia. Shawn, however, also experienced abdominal cramps, mild chest pains, and racing heartbeat until her body adjusted to the medication. If one tricyclic antidepressant doesn't relieve some of your symptoms, it is possible that another one would.

NARDIL

While Nardil is an antidepressant, it is considerably different from the tricyclic antidepressants. It is an MAO inhibitor, which means it inhibits an enzyme called monoamine oxidase. MAO is found in the mitochondria of certain cells (the mitochondria act as the powerhouse of the cell). While the therapeutic effect of Nardil for CFS is still anecdotal, enough interest has been raised so that scientific studies are being undertaken.

The most serious drawback of Nardil is that you can have a hyperpyretic or hypertensive crisis if you mistakenly combine it with certain medicines, foods, or beverages. *Hypertensive crisis* means that your blood pressure increases dramatically; *hyperpyretic crisis* means an exceptionally high fever. These are very dangerous situations, and in extreme cases could be fatal. Therefore, the use of this drug requires strict supervision by a physician, as well as certain dietary restrictions. You need to be aware and well informed. Any substances that contain a high tyramine content must be avoided. These include, but are not limited to, aged foods such as cheese or wine. You also have to be careful about taking certain medications, such as cold tablets, nasal decongestants, and even tryptophan. Your physician can inform you of all the precautions you need to be concerned about when taking Nardil. You should ask your doctor about Procardia, a drug that can quickly bring relief during a hypertensive crisis.

ADENOSINE MONOPHOSPHATE (AMP)

AMP is a naturally occurring body product—a hormone that is used by the body in its energy-producing cycle. The drug form of AMP has been used for years in the treatment of various conditions, but has only recently been tried on patients with CFS. It is believed that in CFS patients, naturally occurring AMP is depleted by whatever virus is causing this syndrome. Therefore, AMP is given in the hopes that it can replace this depleted supply. While it has been used for decades, its use for CFS is new, and reports on it are so far only anecdotal. Some patients have claimed some relief of their symptoms from this drug. This treatment is considered experimental and is not widely available.

AMPLIGEN

Ampligen is a drug that is believed to have the dual properties of being an antiviral and an immune stimulant. Its most recent use has been with AIDS patients, but it has been proposed for use with CFS patients, as well. Clinical data reveal few side effects with the drug, but it is still experimental and more research is needed. As of now, I know of no patients who are on this medication, but have heard that some will be trying it.

VISUALIZATION THERAPY

There are many headings I could have given this section. I could have called it "The Power of Positive Thinking" or even "Natural Healing." Whatever the name, many people find relief of their symptoms through meditation, biofeedback, relaxation, and visualization techniques. There are scores of books dealing with this subject, so I am not going to go into great detail.

The philosophy behind these treatments is that your attitude and beliefs affect your illness. It is believed that people have the ability to influence and alter their state of health, positively or negatively. The stress and strain of everyday existence can suppress the immune system, thereby making the body vulnerable to infection. You can improve your health by eliminating stress, having a positive mental attitude, and visualizing that you are getting well.

Laughter is also believed truly to be good medicine. It is believed that laughter causes the release of chemicals from the brain that help reduce inflammation and ease pain. Norman

Cousins partially attributes his remarkable recovery from cancer to this theory. He put it into practice by watching funny movies, such as old Marx Brothers films.

As we have learned from the placebo effect, the mind is a powerful force. If you create positive mental and emotional images, you may be able to influence your illness. While there are many different techniques, you can visualize your powerful immune system fighting and defeating this helpless infection. Then you should imagine yourself healthy and well. I am not sure how I feel about these types of treatments. I do know that, at the very least, a positive rather than a negative attitude makes coping with this illness a lot easier.

HOMEOPATHY

Homeopathy is a natural healing science that uses natural medicines to help the body heal itself. The whole person is treated, not just the physical body. The medicines used are natural herbs, roots, oils, minerals, vitamins, and so on. These natural medicines are tailored to one's particular symptoms. As with any of the natural healing arts, I do not know if homeopathy is able to cure CFS. I do know, however, that there are people who claim to benefit from some of these methods.

ISOPRINOSINE

Isoprinosine is an immune stimulant that acts on specific antibody (T cell) classes. There has been some research that shows that this drug stimulates lymphocyte response, antibody production, and macrophage response to the EB virus. Isoprinosine is still experimental and, to my knowledge, untried as a treatment for CFS. It is not yet approved by the Food and Drug Administration (FDA), so it is unavailable in this country. The reason I mention this medication is that I have heard of patients who plan to be treated with it in Mexico or Canada. Unfortunately, I have yet to hear of any results, either positive or negative, regarding the ability of this drug to help with CFS.

AGGRESSIVE REST THERAPY (ART)

My father-in-law deserves all the credit for the development of this ingenious therapy. He could see that, though it was painstakingly slow, we did seem to improve gradually as we rested. He observed that it was only after we were confined to the house, literally unable to do anything for a year and a half, that we started regaining our strength.

He also realized that none of the treatments or medications we tried had been able to make us well. And he noted that activity always made us worse—that only by resting were we able to lessen the severity of our symptoms. From this he theorized that since rest lessened the severity of our symptoms, it might also be the key to actually making us well. We were so busy chasing after experimental therapies that we were never able to give our bodies the amount of rest they desperately cried out for.

From this humble beginning arose a unique treatment for CFS—aggressive rest therapy (ART). We were not to do anything other than rest. The concept of ART is not just to rest when you feel horribly ill or even merely to eliminate "pushing." This is a program of aggressive rest. Even when you feel you have a little energy, you should rest. In fact, you should rest all the time.

This is probably the most difficult thing you will ever do. It is not easy to rest aggressively, even for people with CFS who are completely exhausted. Whenever you get a little bit of energy, you want to use it before you lose it. With ART, however, you should not put that energy to use for anything but getting well.

This means that you have to curtail all but the essential activities. You will need help with grocery shopping, errands, preparing meals, laundry, cleaning, and so on. For this you may need the help of family and friends, or may even have to hire someone if you can afford to. You may want to contact the churches in your area; they may be able to suggest someone who can help you for a reasonable fee or even donate their services. I offer further suggestions in the chapter titled "Coping with Your Illness."

In the beginning, it is difficult to rest aggressively because you worry about all the things you think you should be doing. You need to regard resting as you do medication. In order for medicine to be effective, you must take it faithfully. In the same manner, you must be faithful to your resting therapy. In order to do this, you have to disregard the unrealistic expectations imposed on you by others as well as by yourself. You are no longer able to do many, if not most, of the things you used to do. Though you may feel that you have no alternative but to continue pushing yourself beyond your limits, in fact, you do have choices. You decide every day what you will spend your energy and strength on. It is amazing how your life changes once you realize how many choices you truly have.

At the end of three months (the minimum amount of time we give each new therapy) we evaluated the effectiveness of ART. I must admit that both Shawn and I did feel better. I am not going to say that by aggressively resting you will get well. You may, but I have no evidence either way. However, we discovered that our illness was much easier to cope with when we were resting. We found that we were not as irritable and had more to give to our relationship.

I honestly feel that this therapy has been a lifesaver for me. I was beginning to feel like a frayed rope, ready to unravel and snap. Thanks to ART, I feel I have some semblance of a life again.

In addition to the treatments I have described, some people try to alleviate their symptoms with other medications, such as antianxiety drugs, sedatives, muscle relaxants, aspirin, nonnarcotic analgesics, antihistamines, antipyretics for fever, and others. There are also many health products that people try, including Barley Green, Royal Jelly, germanium, coenzyme Q10 and others. This list is not exhaustive by any means. Only you and your doctor can evaluate the effectiveness of these medications in relieving some of your symptoms. Do not try any treatment without consulting your doctor first.

With any treatment, it is difficult to be sure whether you are taking enough medicine for a long enough period of time. Shawn and I usually build up to the safest maximum dosage of anything we try and give a treatment a minimum of three months in which to be effective. Up until now, physicians have not had uniform diagnostic criteria by which to compare their patients with the patients of other researchers. As a result, anecdotal accounts of miraculous cures have often spread, only to have it turn out that the people who got well never even had CFS. By the same token, therapies dismissed in the past as useless for CFS need to be reevaluated because they might have been ineffective for precisely the same reason.

I know I have given you a lot to think about. If you have just recently been diagnosed as having CFS, the choice of treatments may seem overwhelming. Don't rush into any treatment. Discuss all your options with your doctor, weighing the risks against the benefits. Some people with CFS are able to manage their illness without the use of medication. If you cannot, carefully choose the treatment that you are most comfortable with. Do not be discouraged if a treatment does not seem to help; I honestly believe that it is only a matter of time until a permanent cure for CFS is discovered.

6

Coping with Your Illness

Coping with a chronic and debilitating illness requires a great many qualities, not the least of which are patience and perseverance.

Patience enables me to endure the constant and continuous presence of chronic fatigue syndrome. The very problems and emotions I struggled to master yesterday come rushing back today with undiminished intensity. Only by patiently taking each day one day at a time am I able to withstand my unrelenting affliction.

Patience without perseverance, however, is like a gun without bullets. Only patience sustained by perseverance strengthens me to continue a desperate fight in which neither victory nor retreat are options. Though the illness is strong, I must be stronger. I defend myself with patience and perseverance, and while I may feel I am losing some battles, I will yet win the war.

THE POWER OF SELF-ESTEEM

Fortunately, patience and perseverance are not the only weapons in my arsenal. I also have the armor of a healthy self-image. So often a poor self-image is the root of the emotional difficulties people experience with CFS. A poor self-image can be just as debilitating as any physical symptom and can exacerbate negative emotions, such as anger, helplessness, loneliness, self-pity, guilt, depression, and fear.

It is not difficult to understand why CFS is powerful enough to damage even the healthiest self-image. This illness may prevent you from being free and independent. You are no longer able to dictate to your body; it dictates to you. Perhaps you used to base your self-esteem on your accomplishments at work and at play. Now any achievements, even minor ones, may seem few and far between.

If you have a severe case of CFS, you are no longer able to be who you once were. The more you wish your illness would just go away, the harder it will be to cope with. You have to admit to yourself that you have a chronic illness and, until such time as you get well, you will not be who you once were. You must put the past to rest. Grieve over it as you would grieve the loss of a loved one, but then let it go. You need to accept and even respect who you are now. By letting go of the past, you can better cope with the present.

At least for now, you need to build a new self. I knew who the old me was, and I dream of who the healed me will be, but now I have to concentrate on defining the present me. I accomplish this by doing what gives me a sense of fulfillment and purpose now, including activities I barely considered worth undertaking when I was well, such as doing a simple puzzle or growing plants. Your life may have changed, but it is no less significant. You must constantly remind yourself that you are important, and you may have to change some ingrained attitudes about what constitutes self-worth.

Many people define themselves by their employment. When that employment is taken away, so is their identity. You may feel that your life is somehow less worthwhile because you can no longer measure your worth by the fruits of your labors. But a person's worth should not be assessed by the amount of money he has earned. I would much rather be respected for my investment in relationships than for my financial success.

Focus on your inner worth. Who you are is more important than what you do. By enduring this illness, you are developing a depth of character that others may never attain. You may be surprised at the precious qualities that unfold within you: patience, understanding, self-control, empathy, and faith. Enduring pain and suffering may not seem noble at the time, only difficult. But in the end, there can be no greater tribute paid to a person than to say that, with courage and humility, he bore the hardships of his suffering.

Certainly don't let another person ruin your self-esteem. It doesn't matter what anyone else thinks about you or your illness. All that matters is that you realize how strong and brave you truly are. People understand only what they want to understand. Don't waste your precious strength trying to defend your status as a valued member of society.

A sense of competence and accomplishment is also important in maintaining your self-worth. Don't dwell on what you can no longer do; instead focus on what you can. Be realistic about your limitations and avoid setting lofty goals that you can't reach. Undertake small, easily accomplished tasks. If you are not bedridden, you may even consider taking up a small hobby, something that is not too draining but is satisfying.

Another necessary component of self-worth is a sense of belonging. It is a blessing to have supportive family and friends who acknowledge your pain and suffering. Rely on them to help you through this painful time in your life. I know how difficult it is to receive; I much prefer giving. But I have learned to graciously accept the help of others because I would not be able to survive without it.

Even with a loving support system, though, CFS may make it difficult for you to feel you truly belong. Consider contacting one of the CFS organizations listed in Appendix C, to find others with this illness whom you can meet or talk to. It is comforting to be with people who know exactly what you are going through. A good support group can help build self-esteem, dispel fear and anxiety, and provide information and encouragement.

You may also want to consider professional counseling to help you build self-esteem. Some of you may be reticent about seeking professional help because it is difficult for you to be open and honest with a stranger. After the first meeting, however, a counselor is no longer a stranger. In fact, he may seem like a good friend.

UNDERSTANDING

Another weapon in the battle against CFS is understanding. Understanding gives you the wisdom to know your foe and defeat it. I am not referring here to understanding CFS from a medical perspective. Rather, I want you to understand how you work, to identify how this illness affects you physically, mentally, emotionally, and spiritually. Knowing how your illness affects you will move it from the abstract to the specific, making it easier to cope with.

Struggling courageously against the ravages of CFS is not the same as blindly ignoring your body's need for rest. Your body has an innate intelligence. It sends messages that must be heeded, not ignored. Your body is not the enemy; it is merely a victim. You must learn to respect its limitations.

If you are disabled by CFS, the benefits of accepting a

life-style of limited activity are obvious. Unfortunately, it took Shawn and me years before we were willing to accept this new life-style. We tried to ignore the limitations imposed by our illness, but we were left barely hanging by an emotional thread.

We now determine whether or not an activity is worthwhile by how much strength and energy it requires. If it requires more than its potential benefit, it is not worth doing. Learn from our mistake and choose to accept your limitations before you no longer have the choice. Think of being realistic about your limitations not as cowardly surrender, but as a beneficent truce. It is never a sign of weakness to be realistic.

Of course, changing your life-style may be difficult. We spend our entire lives under the shadow of preconceived expectations. When Shawn and I were first married, she assumed it was her ''wifely'' role to cook and clean, and she felt guilty whenever she needed my help. When you're chronically ill, though, preconceived roles become meaningless. Your only expectation should be to rest as much as possible so you have the strength to cope with your illness.

Adapting to a life-style of limited activity requires thought and imagination, as well as the ability to define priorities. To define your priorities, scrutinize every activity and eliminate all but the essential. It wasn't until we started ART (aggressive rest therapy, discussed in the chapter on treatments) that we began to change our thinking from ''But we have to...'' to ''Do we have to...?'' We examined every activity, realized how much of our precious strength was being stolen by unnecessary endeavors, and eliminated all but the most important.

At first we felt selfish for choosing only the activities that were important to us, but we knew it was a physical and emotional necessity. Now we have struck a balance by occasionally doing what others want, even if it is not in our best interest. All in all, though, we have cut down on our activities tremendously. This new life-style keeps us emotionally sane, which is just as important to our health as any medicine. In the process, we have learned many energy-saving tips we would like to pass along to you.

Clothes are incredible energy wasters. Try to wear clothes that don't need ironing. You should also consider using a laundry service if you can afford one. Some laundry services do a very good job and are not prohibitively expensive.

Cleaning the house is also very draining. We contacted a local church that had a program for helping the elderly and disabled. The people who take part in this program donate their services or charge a small fee. If you cannot find such a program, perhaps you could hire a high school student to help around the house.

Try to prepare simple meals. Find out if there is a Meals on Wheels program in your area. This program brings inexpensive meals right to your doorstep. There are also grocery stores and restaurants that will deliver food or meals.

Cleaning up after a meal can be more draining than preparing it. Consider investing in a dishwasher. If that is too expensive, try using as many paper products as you can. It is much easier to throw out a plate than to wash it.

Save yourself from errands by shopping and banking by mail. When we do run errands, we organize them so we can accomplish them all during one outing. We limit using our car to only once or twice a week, forcing us to make better use of our time out. We have to rely on friends and relatives for many of our errands. For example, my parents help with grocery shopping and cooking, as well as taking care of some of our correspondence and phone calls.

We have learned to think of ourselves as a little cup full of life-sustaining water. Any activity, no matter how trivial, depletes us of this water. Since our illness prevents us from refilling the cup, it becomes our responsibility to guard this water as we would guard our life.

COPING WITH YOUR EMOTIONS

The weapon of understanding entails not only knowing your physical limitations, but understanding how CFS affects you emotionally. Every patient with CFS must learn to recognize and cope with many difficult emotions, especially anger, helplessness, loneliness, self-pity, guilt, depression, and fear. These emotions recur with distressing regularity. I want to share some of the painful emotions I struggle with, as well as some of the ways I try to cope with them. CFS is a very demanding illness, but its demands can be met. I hope that this section will help you meet this challenge.

Anger

I used to consider myself a very even-tempered person, slow to anger, slow to lash out. CFS has changed all that. I don't think my basically tranquil personality has been irrevocably altered, but it has undergone some incredible changes. A pool of anger boils and bubbles within me. Without warning, I can erupt like a volcano, incinerating the innocent in my fiery path.

Though CFS is the fundamental source of my anger, it is rarely the recipient. It does no good to get angry at this illness. It cannot be scathed or tempered even by the most emotional outburst.

My angry outbursts are usually triggered by someone or something causing me to expend my energy. Just as a scuba diver's life depends on conserving his oxygen, I must conserve my energy. I become angry when I am forced to waste my strength on useless endeavors. Even something as trivial as being asked to repeat myself can ignite the flames of anger within me. When I am feeling very ill, the slightest irritation can generate the angriest outburst.

I struggle every day merely to survive. I feel as if I am precariously balanced on a tightrope, crossing a deep and deadly gorge. Every ounce of strength is needed just to keep my balance. I lash out in anger because I am afraid of falling. When my defenses are worn down and I feel threatened, my instincts take over. I attack before being attacked.

Frustration is a key component of anger, and my illness is a constant source of frustration. Each frustration that is ignored or denied festers along with other suppressed frustrations. The person who is responsible for causing the latest frustration, the one that breaks the camel's back, receives my outpouring of wrath.

My anger can range from simple annoyance to vindictive outrage, but it usually burns itself out quickly. I find that the key to successfully coping with anger is releasing it. Don't suppress it. Anger is a natural and inevitable part of life. It is as normal an emotion as happiness; it just happens to be a lot louder.

In order to vent anger safely and healthily, it is important to identify the source of that anger. Obviously, CFS is the fundamental source, but it is rarely the immediate cause. If you do not identify the proper cause of your anger, you run the risk of misdirecting it. Inevitably, the target of misdirected anger will be the people who deserve it the least—your loved ones.

The tendency to lash out at others is greatly increased when we are very ill. We feel out of control and helpless. We may need to feel that we still have an impact on someone else's life, even if that impact is angry and hurtful, even if the people we hurt are people we love. Anger may also be purposely self-destructive. By hurting those closest to us, we also hurt ourselves. We punish others in order to punish ourselves.

Perhaps we have a hard time expressing our need for attention, so we grab it in any way we can. Or we may lash out in anger at our loved ones simply because we are afraid. We may be fearful that we are no longer lovable and that our loved ones may desert us. We hurt them because we fear they are going to hurt us. This can become a self-fulfilling prophecy: Our hurtful behavior ends up making us unlovable.

Anger may be caused by an insensitive friend who pretends to believe your illness is real but obviously has doubts. Or maybe you are expected to do something that is beyond your ability. Perhaps you are angry because you have been sick for so very long. Whatever the reasons, our loved ones do not deserve to be the recipients of our venom. Only by recognizing the source of our anger can we avoid misdirecting it and lashing out at others.

Try to be aware of your emotions, right from the first moment you start to feel angry. The old saw of counting to ten really does work. It gives you a chance to think about what you are doing. If you are able, use that time to do an emotional self-evaluation. Look at the situation objectively. We often become needlessly angry because we think we have been wronged in some way, when in fact it is our perception that is wrong.

My wife has a loving and gentle spirit, and is always quick to consider the other person's point of view. That used to drive me crazy. I didn't want to see the other person's side or give him the benefit of the doubt. I wanted only to be mad! The more she taught me about the gracious art of compassionate understanding, however, the more I realized how truly rare righteous indignation is.

Once you become attuned to identifying the cause of your anger, you should try to avoid those situations that are most likely to make you angry. Many such situations are unavoidable, of course, but even they will be easier to deal with if you eliminate the ones you can. I have found that ignoring my own limitations is the greatest provocation of anger. When I push myself to the point of exhaustion, I no longer have the strength to control my anger.

Finally, learn to be forgiving, not only of others but of yourself as well. People are fallible; we all make mistakes. Share your feelings with those you love. If you are hurt by someone, talk it out. Don't hold grudges. A grudge doesn't hurt the person you are angry with; it only hurts you.

Helplessness

It is not easy to be seen as helpless in a society that prides itself on its go-it-alone mentality. Rugged individualism, not helpless dependence, is what is respected and admired. The need for others is disdained as a sign of weakness rather than acknowledged as a natural consequence of being human.

I don't have the option of blindly ignoring my humanness. My illness is a constant reminder of how terribly frail and vulnerable I am. Sometimes I am not even certain I can continue the fight—to bravely and stoically endure. And in our society, gold medals are given for winning the race, not for merely struggling to stay in it.

You may no longer be able to do the things you want or may no longer have the strength to do the things you need. If you have a severe case of CFS, you may be totally dependent on the help and support of others, physically and emotionally. At best, you feel like an invalid, unable to take care of your basic needs.

Needing others, however, does not make you any less of a person. Needing and being needed are as basic to humanity as breathing or eating. Those who pride themselves on walking alone through life deprive themselves of one of the greatest joys of living.

You may also feel weak and helpless because you are unable to influence your recovery. But remember: Recovering from an illness requires no great feat of strength; your body is designed to do that naturally and unconsciously. What does require incredible inner strength is enduring a chronic illness. Helpless people do not endure chronic illness—they succumb to it.

You deserve admiration, not derision, for what you endure. Many people with CFS have humbly learned to endure a level of pain and sickness that would devastate a healthy person. And considering the cultural values we were all raised with, it takes a lot more strength and courage to ask others for help than it does to suffer silently—and needlessly—alone.

Loneliness

Loneliness may be the most prevalent emotional problem among Americans today, and this is especially true of people who suffer with CFS. I can be in a room full of people and feel totally alone, completely isolated by this illness. I often feel as if I am on the outside of life looking in, no longer sharing any common interests with the rest of society. Forced out of the world of health and activity, I have been dragged into a world of sickness and pain. I have joined a different brotherhood of humanity, the brotherhood of suffering.

It is natural to feel lonely when you are chronically ill. People with CFS can't help but feel different from most other people. The more intense this feeling, the more difficult it is to reach out to others. Your healthy friends may not visit anymore because they feel uncomfortable, not knowing what to say or what to do. You get tired of having to explain your illness all the time, and after a while, it just seems easier to be alone.

To deal with loneliness, you must first decide that you don't want to be alone. I am not referring here to solitude. I love being alone when it is my choice. Loneliness is a feeling of total isolation. You may have physical proximity to other people, but no emotional contact.

It is not easy reaching out to others when you are chronically ill. There is an inherent fear of rejection. You may fear that people won't accept you because you are ill. Or perhaps you are afraid they won't accept you because they don't believe you are ill. You must confront these fears head-on. Unfortunately, you cannot avoid meeting insensitive people, but you can't let them prevent you from reaching out to others.

One of the best ways to combat loneliness is meeting with other people who have CFS. You can derive comfort from the realization that you are not alone. There are thousands of people who have the same illness you do. I have been at support group meetings where new members burst into tears of relief because they had finally met someone who knew what they were going through.

Empathy eliminates loneliness. If there is no support group in your area, you can at least talk to someone with CFS over the phone. I have had many phone conversations with fellow patients. While it is not as personal as meeting them, just talking seemed to help a lot. You can also meet with people who have other serious or chronic illnesses. Even though they may not know some of the specific trials you experience with CFS, they can still be empathetic and caring.

Finally, try to be the kind of person others enjoy being with. If you are continually angry or feeling sorry for yourself, no one is going to want to spend time with you. Don't make other people feel guilty for being well. If you are envious of the health of your friends, you will drive them away. It is a safe bet that if you are the type of person others enjoy being with, you will not be lonely for very long.

Self-Pity

Self-pity is an emotion we are often unable to recognize within ourselves. It so warps our perceptions that we cannot look at ourselves objectively. Often we don't want to deal with this emotion because, in small doses, it makes us feel better. Initially, it even gains us sympathy from the people around us. But self-pity is like a drug; it may make us feel better temporarily, but the price we pay is too costly. People who feel sorry for themselves are miserable to be around. They are unable to care for anyone other than themselves, and soon there is no one left to care *but* themselves.

Isolated by your own self-involvement, you will see yourself as an undeserving victim, which will only compound your misery. Your self-pity will intensify as each new perceived injustice leaves you feeling betrayed. Eventually, people will think that you are doing such a good job generating sympathy on your own that you don't need any help. The sympathy you are so desperately trying to engender will never be given.

My greatest struggle against self-pity comes when I compare myself to other people. I feel as if they have everything in the world and I have nothing. All of our friends and relatives are buying houses and cars. Some are graduating from school, while others are receiving job promotions. Many are having children, and all of them make more money than Shawn and I do. Their lives are totally fulfilling, and mine is totally empty. They are incredibly happy, while I am incredibly miserable.

Actually, very little of what I have just written is true. But when you are feeling sorry for yourself, you lose the ability to separate truth from projection. Sure, most of our friends are buying houses and having children, and all of them make more money than we do. But their lives are not picture perfect. They have problems of their own. Neither is my life totally void. I have a loving wife, caring friends, a supportive family, and a faithful Lord.

It is normal to feel sorry for yourself once in a while, but if you are not careful, self-pity could easily turn into resentment. Rather than sharing in the lives and successes of your friends and relatives, you could become envious and bitter, walking around with a chip on your shoulder. Thinking that you were somehow cheated in this life, you would blame everyone and everything for your misfortune. In short, you would become your own worst enemy, for these destructive attitudes would separate you from the love and support you so desperately need.

You may consider the old adage "Count your blessings" to be merely a cliché. Perhaps you feel that your blessings could be counted on one finger! If you are honest with yourself, though, I am sure you could name quite a few blessings in your life.

Finally, find someone you can openly and honestly share your feelings with. It isn't necessary for them to have CFS to be supportive. Although Rita, one of Shawn's closest friends, is healthy and lives halfway across the country, they made a commitment to call each other every couple of weeks. Shawn derives strength and encouragement just from knowing how much she cares.

I don't talk to my Aunt Kaye in Florida as often as Shawn talks with Rita, but she is my source of encouragement. She has suffered what seems to be a lifetime of crippling rheumatoid arthritis, but her spirit is as gentle and loving as when she was well. In comparison to her suffering, my illness is minor, yet she has never made me feel that way. She knows the agony of illness better than anyone, and the example of her life is my source of inspiration.

Guilt

You cannot suffer the life-altering impact of CFS without also suffering feelings of guilt. It seems to be around every corner ready to pounce. Guilt comes from many different sources. You may feel guilty because you can no longer fulfill your obligations to your family, take proper care of the children, or bring home a paycheck. Whatever the circumstances, CFS prevents people from fulfilling many of their normal roles and obligations. This invariably leads to pangs of guilt.

You may even feel guilty due to the illness itself. You know you need to talk about your struggles, yet you may feel guilty doing so because CFS is not an illness that most people understand. You may not look severely ill, and you don't want to sound like a complainer. Or you may be wondering if you are somehow responsible for becoming ill. Perhaps you failed to take your health seriously enough, or didn't pay attention when your body was pleading with you for rest.

Whatever the reason, guilt is a destructive emotion that should not be regarded lightly. It eats away at you, making you feel weak, inadequate, and insecure. Guilt often stems from being too critical and unforgiving of yourself. It helps to realize that the perceived source of guilt is usually unfounded. For example, you may believe that you are ill because God is punishing you, but this guilt is based on an inaccurate understanding of God. Another source of guilt may be your inability to do the things you believe you are supposed to do. Again, these feelings are based on unrealistic expectations of your health and, quite possibly, an unrealistic assessment of what your family truly expects of you.

Share your feelings with those around you. You may be surprised to learn that you are the only one who expects so much of yourself. If others do expect more than you can give, they may be unaware of the severity of your illness. Don't assume that most people are sensitive enough to realize the true state of your health. I have found that I have to verbalize and demonstrate the severity of my affliction before people will understand.

Examine the source of your guilt. Try to determine if mistaken perceptions or unrealistic expectations are the actual source of the problem. If you find that the source of your guilt is other people, discuss it with them. They may be projecting their own feelings of inadequacy and guilt onto you.

Finally, do not be preoccupied with thoughts of retribution or punishment. Don't be obsessed with looking backward, trying to determine why you became ill. All that matters now is that you are ill. Spend your energy constructively, trying to cope with this disease.

Depression

Depression, that abject feeling of total despair and futility, is often the result of the suppression of other emotions, such as guilt and anger. Often when CFS victims look back over the course of their illness and see how very long they have been suffering—then look forward and find no relief in sight—a tidal wave of depression comes rushing over them, threatening to drown them in a sea of despair.

When I experience depression, I am able to see only the negatives in my life. Nothing is going right, and living is more a burden than a blessing. I am tired of being sick and sick of being tired. I am frustrated because I am unable to do the things I want and, more important, I am unable to be the type of person I want to be. Totally helpless and defeated by this disease, I have lost almost everything that is of value to me: my ability to work and provide for my family, my ability to be the husband Shawn deserves, my freedom, my health, and my ability to serve God as a minister.

Forced to look into the very abyss of my own mortality, I feel stretched to the absolute limits of my emotional and physical ability to endure. But just when I reach my breaking point, I discover something truly remarkable: an ability to endure beyond what I thought was my limit. This is not something I am quick to take credit for; I feel more like an astonished bystander watching this miraculous display.

This ability to survive is not unique to me. When you are overcome with depression and have reached the end of your endurance, encourage yourself that you can endure. Any limits you perceive are just that: perceived. There *are* no limits to your ability to endure. You can, and must, endure the trials of this illness.

It is important to make the distinction between depression and discouragement. Discouragement is the temporary feeling you have when you fail or are defeated. Depression is a long-term emotional state of total dejection. It distorts your thinking, which can make it difficult to recognize when depression is beginning. But as soon as you do realize it, remember that most of your thoughts and emotions will be distorted.

Avoid making any major decisions when you feel depressed. Depression is like a long, dark tunnel. You may not see the light at the end of the tunnel, but it is there. Be patient and you will soon be out of the darkness and into the light.

It is critical that depression not be allowed to build to the point that you harbor suicidal thoughts. Many people with CFS have, at one point or another, considered suicide. I doubt anyone could suffer with this syndrome without entertaining the idea at least once. When you are deeply depressed, however, you are incapable of thinking clearly and rationally. Find someone to talk to if you are struggling with feelings of suicide. Don't be ashamed or embarrassed; get professional help.

Remember also that depression is an actual symptom of this syndrome, perhaps even caused chemically. So merely trying to change your mental attitude may not have a noticeable effect. If you are suffering from severe depression, consult your doctor immediately. There are antidepressant medications that may help.

Again, learning to accept the limitations of your illness may help prevent depression. Don't be self-critical; rather, learn the art of self-loving and forgiving. People who have a hard time liking themselves fall more easily into the clutches of depression.

When you feel depressed, reinforce positive behavior and change your environment or routine. Open the shades and let the sun shine in. Turn the TV off and go for a short walk, breathing the fresh air. Listen to joyful or soothing music, or take a warm bubble bath. Maybe you should even consider getting a pet. Treat yourself by doing things that make you happy. Above all, reach out to others for help. Talk about your discouragement and vent your feelings with a good cry. Don't dwell on the past or worry about the future; just try to get through today.

Fear

It is understandable if CFS makes you anxious. Sometimes I am afraid to meet new people because I am self-conscious about my illness. Even though I have learned to expect them, I still dread the looks of doubt and disbelief. It is a universal weakness of mankind to worry about what other people may think.

I am also afraid of the effects my illness may have on my body. No one knows the long-term effects of CFS. I wonder if I am more susceptible to other diseases, or whether this illness will make me weaker than I already am. I wonder if the medications I have taken will do more harm than good. I am afraid of the future—that I may never be well enough to have children or to complete my seminary training. Contemplating questions that have no easy answers invariably leads to worry and to fear.

General feelings of apprehension and concern are a natural result of being chronically ill, but intense feelings of dread and paralyzing anxiety are not normal. You may feel afraid because you feel threatened and helpless, but you can't allow these feelings to ruin your life. You can't let your fear of people's disbelief prevent you from living. You can't let your fear of medications prevent you from trying safe treatments that might make you well. And you can't let your fears of the effects of your illness prevent you from living as well as you can with that illness.

If your biggest fear is that you may be developing some illness even more threatening than CFS, tell your physician. He can provide the testing necessary to reassure you of where you stand. If your anxiety is that you may be shunned by friends and colleagues who have heard through the grapevine that you are sick with some mysterious illness, the best thing you can do is talk openly with them. Explain what they need to know about CFS. Reassure them that they are in no danger.

Support groups are the best way I know to conquer anxiety. They allow you to express your fears and concerns to others who are dealing with those same feelings. Sharing and confronting fear is the best way I know to dispel it. But if, after sharing your feelings with your peers, you still feel overwhelmed with anxiety, I strongly urge you to seek professional help.

I realize that all this "good advice" has only limited value to those of you who are too sick to act on it. I also know that when you are suffering, encouragement and advice often seem shallow and worthless. No matter what I write, or how much your family and friends may love you, you still face your pain alone. My only hope is that this chapter encourages you by showing that, while you suffer alone, you are not alone in your suffering. There are others who know what you are going through.

Remember that there is no right way of coping with CFS. We all maintain our balance in different ways. My chief coping mechanism is limited avoidance. I put off dealing with things that I am unable to handle. This allows me to postpone until tomorrow what I am unable to face today.

Some people cope by denying their illness, while others are constantly concerned about it. At different times, you might have to change your coping mechanisms to learn what is effective in a given situation. Sometimes you may need to go with the flow, while other times you need to be contemplative and rational. At times you may deny and avoid your illness, and other times you may prefer to be actively involved. Sometimes you may withdraw from people, while other times you may want to interact with people, behaving as if you were healthy.

All you can do is take each hour one hour at a time. Do whatever is necessary to help you through that hour. If your illness is less severe than mine, coping may not be as difficult as I have depicted. If your illness is more severe, it may actually be more difficult. If you continue to have problems coping with CFS, seek professional help.

And finally, remember to weep when you need to weep, for a false sense of stoic strength only leads us to stiffen and break rather than soften and bend. And share your pain with others, for only a false sense of pride would insist on bearing this most terrible of burdens alone.

7

Overcoming
Financial Hardship

This book would not be complete without addressing one of the greatest health risks facing the chronically ill: financial hardship. Why is that a health risk? Because the fear of financial hardship can coerce the chronically ill to continue working at their jobs even though the strain of employment is literally making them ill. Often, quitting is never even considered because they mistakenly believe that they have no financial alternatives.

It took me a very long time to admit to myself that my illness was not going to go away—that until such time as a cure was discovered, I would be disabled. But eventually it became painfully obvious that even the slightest activity made me feel terribly ill and that continuing my education or holding down a job was impossible.

Now, unless you are independently wealthy (or no longer care about eating), you cannot just decide one day that you are no longer going to work. Since there was every chance I was going to be sick for quite some time, I had to make other financial arrangements. I desperately needed Medicare to cover the expense of treatments, which ran into tens of thousands of dollars. Also, Shawn and I were getting married and needed some way of supporting ourselves. We didn't want to be a financial burden on our parents, making them go into long-term debt, so we followed the only logical course left open to us. We applied for disability benefits.

Making the decision to take Social Security benefits was not a monumental step for me; admitting that I was not getting better was much more difficult. I welcomed disability benefits with gratitude rather than humiliation because they allowed me to rest, giving me the only chance I had of living with my illness.

Though I am on disability, I understand why the thought of receiving financial aid may be difficult for some of you. Your self-esteem may be tied to your job or to how much money you earn, making the prospect of being on disability, with a subsequent loss of income, too much to bear. Maybe you resent the loss of self-sufficiency that receiving aid implies. Perhaps accepting disability means admitting that you are sick and can no longer hold on to your hopes and dreams; you feel as if you are giving up and giving in to your illness.

Though I can empathize with those feelings, I would still encourage you to consider applying for benefits if working is hurting your health. My hope is that you will avoid the mistake I made. I ruined my health because I was afraid to concede that I might not overcome my illness. Rather than think that you have no financial alternative but to work, at least consider the possibility that you may have no other *health* alternative but to stop.

I can't promise that you won't have to make some sacrifices, or even that once you quit your job you are assured of receiving benefits. But if I have learned one fundamental truth from this illness, it is that there is nothing on this earth as precious as your health. Without it, you are unable to function on any level: spiritually, socially, emotionally, mentally, or physically. You need to guard it as jealously as you do your life, for if you ruin your health by pushing yourself unwisely, you run the risk of wasting your life.

We live in a wonderful country that has emergency provisions for people in need. For years, your tax dollars have been hard at work providing for others who are less fortunate than yourself. These same dollars have also been set aside, in the form of Social Security and many other programs, against the event that you should ever become disabled.

I know that for some of you, the prospect of taking government aid is distasteful. You may hold the misconception that any government program is a form of charity. I don't. I look on it as an insurance policy that my family has contributed to over their entire lifetimes. By paying Social Security and other taxes, we have provided not only for our retirement, but for times of hardship as well.

My father-in-law has calculated that if he had taken all the Social Security taxes he has paid to the government and invested them wisely over the past thirty years, he would be able to support my wife and me with thousands of dollars a month for the rest of our lives. The sweat and hard labor that go into paying taxes entitle you to receive benefits. You wouldn't consider disability benefits from a private insurance company to be charity. In a very real sense, the government is just the largest insurer in the country.

The only factor, then, that should determine whether you apply for disability benefits is the extent of your disability. I won't pretend that the application process is easy, but by explaining the major programs, and by guiding you through some of the problems you might encounter in applying, I hope to make the process as painless as possible.

EMPLOYEE BENEFITS

The very first step you should take is to speak with your employer and find out if your company provides disability benefits. Frequently, companies do offer disability insurance for their employees, and these benefits are typically much easier to obtain than Social Security. Your personnel director or supervisor can explain how to apply.

SOCIAL SECURITY

If your company has no disability provisions, you should go to your local Social Security office to apply for benefits. Never assume, for any reason, that you are ineligible. I was told by a hospital social worker that I was not entitled to benefits because I was a student and because my illness was not considered disabling. Fortunately, I have a persistent spirit and I refused to believe there wasn't some form of government aid to help people in my situation.

Eligibility Requirements

There are only two requirements you must meet in order to receive disability benefits. The first is that you be totally disabled, unable to perform even sedentary work. The second is that you have paid some Social Security taxes five out of the last ten years. This is a general rule and there are exceptions. Go to your local Social Security office for more details. Students may also be eligible because Social Security taxes were probably withheld from their salaries during summer employment.

Eligibility for disability benefits is not based on your income or assets. If, for some reason, you do not meet the two requirements, do not despair. You may still be eligible for financial aid in the form of welfare assistance, rental subsidy programs, Medicaid, or food stamps. These programs are discussed later in this chapter.

Your First Visit

When you go to the Social Security office, you will be assigned a caseworker. The caseworker will have a record of your work history as well as a record of the amount you have paid in Social Security taxes. You must make sure that their records are correct because the amount of your monthly benefits depends in part on the amount of taxes you have paid.

Once you have determined that you have paid Social Security taxes and are eligible to apply, the next step is proving that you are disabled. Unfortunately, this is not the easiest of tasks. Unlike our judicial system, where you are considered innocent until proven guilty, at Social Security you are assumed to be able to work. It is up to you to prove you are not. If you are aware of this in advance, you will not be as easily discouraged if you are rejected and have to appeal. If you are patient and persistent, there is every likelihood that, in the end, you will be approved.

Your caseworker will explain what you must do to file your initial application. It was my good fortune to have a caring and concerned caseworker who did not make me feel like a second-class citizen. But I have run into caseworkers who couldn't care less about me or my illness. Don't be intimidated by heartless caseworkers. Fortunately, they are not the people who decide your case.

Discussing your disability with a stranger can be embarrassing, especially since people with CFS often look so much better than they feel. Don't minimize the extent of your illness or the traumatic impact it has on your life just because you are afraid of sounding like a complainer. The only way Social Security can make a fair decision is if you let them have all the facts. When you are asked questions about your physical limitations, answer according to a typical day, not one of your better ones. Don't forget the particularly horrible days when you feel absolutely wretched. Patiently and accurately explain your disability to the caseworker. Don't exaggerate, but don't minimize.

Wading through this sea of bureaucratic red tape may make the Social Security system seem designed to be as discouraging as possible. Perhaps this is in response to all the attention that has recently been focused on the minority of people who abuse the system.

Whatever the reason, I don't think Social Security has always been this intimidating. This change in attitude can be seen by comparing the old and new Social Security cards. My card, issued in the late sixties, politely informs me what to do should I ever lose my card or change my name. It says that when I reach age sixty-two, or if I am ever unable to work because of a disability, I should contact my local Social Security office. It even encourages me to inquire about retirement checks. To top it off, it invites me to sign up for Medicare when I reach sixty-two, even if I am not yet ready to retire. You get the impression that they really do want to help.

That's not the feeling you get reading my wife's Social Security card, which is only a few years old because her name changed when we were married. First comes a warning: "Do not laminate this card!" Then it says that the card is invalid if it is not signed. It proceeds to threaten her, saying that if she improperly uses the card she can be thrown in prison and fined. She is then reminded that the card is the property of Social Security and must be returned to them whenever they request it. Finally, at the very bottom of the card, they get around to the reason she even has it in the first place. They inform her that she should contact Social Security for any other matter. Are they kidding? After all that, I'd be afraid even to touch their card, let alone contact one of their offices!

All kidding aside, if you are prepared for the frustration of a long and difficult process, you will not be one of the people discouraged from receiving their benefits. In the end, when all the paperwork is finished, the system does provide for those who persevere. But you must be prepared for an incredibly invasive investigation. By the time they're finished, it will seem as if Social Security knows everything there is to know about you and a little more. From your finances to your medical records, they will leave no stone unturned.

The Initial Application

When you file your initial application, you will be asked many different questions, even some that seem to have no bearing on your illness. You will be asked how much you can lift, how far you can walk, how long you can sit, and so on. You will also be asked about the nature of your disability and why you are unable to work.

When answering these questions, be as specific as possible. Don't just tell them that you have chronic fatigue syndrome and expect them to understand. Tell them the ins and outs of your illness. You must prove not only that you are unable to perform your previous job, but that you are unable to perform any job, including sedentary labor. If you are completely disabled by your illness, explain that you can't walk, sit, or stand except for brief periods. Discuss your fatigue, your aches and pains, your mental impairment, and how you are affected when you try to work. Tell them how difficult it is just trying to do the chores around the house, how even the simple tasks of personal hygiene are draining.

Medical Documentation

You will be asked to provide all your medical records, as well as specific medical evidence to support your claim. Social Security will contact your doctors directly to obtain their opinion of your disability. Do not assume that a simple statement that you are disabled will be enough to win your case. You need letters from your doctors that clearly and specifically explain why you are unable to do any type of work.

The letter below is not the one I used when I applied, but it is much like the one I would use today. Show it to your doctors to use as a guide, though of course some of the specifics mentioned, for example acyclovir, do not apply to every patient. Your letter(s) should be tailored to your specific circumstances.

Social Security Administration
Bureau of Disability Determination

To Whom It May Concern:

I am writing to certify that Jane Doe is completely disabled for performance of even sedentary tasks due to the following debilitating conditions.

Jane Doe has undergone detailed sophisticated medical and immunologic evaluations and physical examinations which, along with my long-term treatment of the patient, since March 1987, constitute the basis for my professional conclusions.

Jane Doe has been suffering the effects of chronic fatigue syndrome, formerly known as chronic Epstein-Barr virus, and mild hypogammaglobulinemia. Individuals so infected as Ms. Doe have severely disabling symptoms of fatigue, malaise, recurrent pharyngitis, cervical and inguinal adenopathy, arthralgia, lethargy, weakness, and low-grade fever. She is also seriously debilitated by the following neurological symptoms: dizziness, headaches, mental fogging, confusion, and an inability to think clearly or concentrate. These symptoms have persisted since their onset in February 1986 and, due to the degree of their severity, have rendered her totally disabled.

Following the diagnostic guidelines for chronic fatigue syndrome established by Holmes et al. in the March 1988 *Annals of Internal Medicine,* Ms. Doe has undergone sophisticated tests to rule out any other possible diseases. Laboratory findings indicate the following immune abnormalities which are consistent with what we find in other CFS patients: Ms. Doe exhibits suppressed activity of natural killer cells. She has also undergone Epstein-Barr virus serology titer tests which reveal persistently abnormal antibody titers to selected Epstein-Barr virus antigens. While they are no longer considered diagnostic, these tests indicate an abnormal immune response. She has also undergone immunoglobulin subclass tests which reveal partial immunoglobulin deficiency. Physical examinations reveal shotty nodes in the posterior cervical and inguinal areas.

Ms. Doe's historical, clinical, serologic, and immunologic findings are entirely consistent with the diagnosis of chronic fatigue syndrome.

In the summer of 1987, Ms. Doe received a trial of several weeks of intravenous and oral acyclovir. She also received intravenous gamma globulin treatments for over a year, beginning in November 1987. Other empiric trials include Indocin, vitamin therapy, Diamox, Pamelor, Sinequan, Nardil, and high doses of vitamin C, all without significant or sustained benefits. She has also tried alternative therapies such as acupuncture, chiropractic care, and special diets without improvement.

Jane Doe is capable of standing, walking, carrying, lifting, and doing sedentary tasks while sitting down only sporadically or for an insignificant amount of time. She needs to rest between activities. Jane Doe is unable to perform even a sedentary job part-time. Chronic fatigue syndrome has severely limited both her physical and mental capacity to perform even basic activities. Her neurological symptoms render any activity requiring concentration, including reading and driving, very difficult. She is capable of only mild activity on an intermittent basis. Most days, she may be able to do no more than wash, dress, and prepare meals. On other days, she may be able to take care of correspondence or do some light reading. Her ability to sustain any activity for more than a few hours a day is unpredictable, and any prolonged activity (even sedentary activity) worsens her condition and could cause exacerbation of her symptoms.

Ms. Doe has unsuccessfully attempted low stress exercise and activities many times, but, as for most people with this syndrome, any activity results in a worsening of her symptoms. Restricting activity is, at present, the only way to prevent exacerbation of the symptoms.

I have had experience in evaluating and treating many patients with CFS. The fatigue these patients suffer with is unlike the normal fatigue experienced by healthy individuals. It is a profound weakness that makes simple tasks such as brushing their teeth seem overwhelming. Although individuals with this syndrome frequently do not appear significantly ill, most are, in fact, markedly disabled and frequently unable to be gainfully employed.

Patients are typically young or middle-aged adults who fail to fully recover clinically and immunologically from acute viral infection. Detailed observations have been reported by: Holmes, et al. in ''Chronic Fatigue Syndrome: A Working Case Definition.'' (*Annals of Internal Medicine,* 1988; 108:387–389).

In conclusion, I do not know whether Jane Doe's disability is likely to resolve. Very few chronic fatigue syndrome patients have experienced spontaneous improvement. There is no known cure or medication which is effective in treating this syndrome and since

Ms. Doe has not experienced any relief from the best available therapies, it is my opinion that she will continue to be disabled and unable to be employed in any manner for an indeterminate period of time.

I will be following Jane Doe in the near future and will continue other forms of investigational therapy to counteract the ravages of chronic fatigue syndrome.

If I can be of any further help in the support of Jane Doe's application for disability benefits, please don't hesitate to call on me.

Sincerely,

M. J. Leavay, M.D.

Any letters your doctors write should at least be as detailed and specific as the one above. It must stress that you are unable to do any type of work, including sedentary tasks, and the reasons why (for example, that activity worsens your condition). It should also explain the nature of your illness as well as your symptoms, and should validate the severity of your illness, especially regarding the limitations it imposes. Social Security will believe your limitations only if they are validated by a doctor. If your doctor can prove that you have an immune deficiency or some other ailment as well as CFS, your chances of being accepted may be improved. I would strongly encourage you to give your doctor a copy of the article "Social Security Disability Assessment: Inseparable from Patient Care," by Douglas M. Smith (see Appendix D). It gives physicians all the information they need to know in order to write an effective letter.

If you have more than one doctor, have each of them write a letter. Since doctors' letters are one of the most important ways you have of proving you are disabled, it is important that you keep seeing your doctors regularly. Notify them that they will soon be contacted by Social Security. Any delay on their part in sending your records or writing their opinions slows down the process.

At this point, you have the option of informing your senators or congressmen that you have applied for Social Security. They have no influence to help you win your case, but they will let the Social Security office know they are interested in the results of your application. At the very least, this special interest should help keep your claim from being delayed or getting lost. In other words, Social Security is being held accountable by an elected official.

After your initial application is finally done, your medical evidence submitted, and your representatives contacted, all that is left to do is wait for Social Security's decision. This will take weeks or even months. When that fateful day does arrive, do not be discouraged if your initial application was rejected. Social Security does now recognize CFS (as of this writing Social Security refers to this syndrome as chronic Epstein-Barr virus) as a legitimate disabling condition, but proving you have CFS and that you are disabled is not always easy. Social Security forwarded my first rejection to our nation's research hospital, the National Institutes of Health, where I was having experimental drugs pumped into my veins in an effort to overcome this illness. It didn't seem to matter to Social Security that this was obviously the action of someone who was truly ill.

The First Appeal

If you are rejected, the second stage of your disability application is the appeal for reconsideration. This is very similar to the first stage. You have to fill out more forms and submit additional evidence to support your claim. The person who decides your case at this point still has very strict guidelines to follow, but does have more flexibility. In other words, he can be more lenient when making his determination.

The chances of being approved for chronic fatigue syndrome

during the first two applications have increased dramatically since I first became ill, but do not be discouraged if you are once again rejected. You can appeal this rejection as well. When I applied, this syndrome was totally unknown, and I knew that in all likelihood I would be rejected. Therefore, I regarded the initial application, as well as the appeal for reconsideration, as something to be dispensed with quickly. The sooner I could get this over with, I felt, the sooner I could move on to the second appeal—the appeal that made a difference.

The Second Appeal

This second appeal is decided by an administrative law judge. Pleading your cause before a judge sounds more ominous than it is. Your hearing is not held in a court, but in an office. This hearing is where you make or break your case. Since it is such an important meeting, I recommend that you retain an attorney. It is a sad commentary on our society that the disabled and needy have to hire a lawyer just to secure what is rightfully theirs. For some reason, however, your chances of winning are increased when you hire a lawyer.

Make sure that you retain a lawyer who has experience with Social Security hearings. They typically work for a percentage of the retroactive benefits you receive if you win your case. Retroactive benefits are the accumulated monthly benefits you would have received all along had your initial application been accepted. If you were disabled for at least a year prior to filing your initial application, you may also be entitled to benefits for some of the months before you applied. Your Social Security caseworker can explain all the rules and requirements as well as calculate the retroactive benefits you are entitled to. If you cannot afford to pay an attorney a percentage of your retroactive benefits, you should contact your Social Security office or the local Legal Aid Society. They may know of lawyers who donate their services.

If one of your doctors is able to attend the hearing, your chances of winning could be greatly increased. His presence will have greater influence than a letter alone. Remember to compensate him for his time. Our doctor, Dr. Oleske, was so kind he wouldn't even send us a bill, so we presented him with a briefcase to thank him for his support.

The administrative law judge is going to ask you many questions. The following list contains some of the questions most frequently asked:

1. You will be asked to give your age, height, and weight and to tell if you are right-handed or left-handed.

2. You will be asked about your marital status, educational background, military record, and any special vocational training you have had.

3. You will be asked about your last job and how much lifting and bending it required. You will also be asked about the last day you worked and what prevented you from returning to work.

4. You will be asked if you can dress and feed yourself, as well as about any impairments you might have. You will be asked if you can perform housework, cooking, laundry, and shopping.

5. You will be asked how far you can walk and run, if you can touch the floor with your hands, and how long you can sit and stand comfortably.

6. You will be asked if you are able to drive a car and, if not, how you got to the hearing.

7. You will be asked about your social contacts: if you visit friends, attend church, have any hobbies, or belong to any clubs or organizations.

8. You will be asked about your typical day: what time you get up, if you watch TV, and how much you sleep.

9. You may be asked about future vocational training, and a vocational expert may be called in to determine if you can be trained to perform some job other than the one you had.

10. You will be asked about your aches and pains. You will be asked to explain, in your own words, how your illness prevents you from working. You will also be asked to describe any medications or treatments you are taking or have tried.
11. On a scale of one to ten, you will be asked to describe the level of pain you experience with and without medication. You will be asked how often you see a doctor.
12. Finally, you will be allowed to tell the judge anything that wasn't already covered regarding your illness.

This list of questions may seem intimidating, but don't be afraid. Think about your answers. During the hearing, answer all the questions clearly and carefully. Once again, don't minimize your illness. The judge needs to know exactly what you are going through. Finally, try not to be too nervous. The majority of people I know who have applied for disability benefits have won. As CFS receives more publicity, benefits should also become easier to obtain.

The Appeals Council

There is a council, called the Appeals Council, that has the final say on all Social Security claims. This means that they have the power not only to grant you benefits even if the administrative law judge denies them, but to *deny* your claim even if the administrative law judge *approved* it. They might do the former if they feel that the law judge was unfair in deciding your case, and they might do the latter if they feel he was not critical enough. It is unusual, however, for the Appeals Council to overturn a favorable decision.

If you are denied benefits, it will probably mean one of two things: either you are not totally disabled, or you have not presented strong enough medical evidence to prove your case. If the administrative law judge denies your claim, you can request your case be heard by the Appeals Council. Make sure you give them conclusive evidence of your disability, with very supportive doctors' letters. If it was the Appeals Council that denied your claim, your case will probably be sent back to the administrative law judge for review. In this case, the same advice applies—submit strong, conclusive evidence and doctors' letters. If after all this you are still denied, and you firmly believe you are disabled, you have only two recourses. One is to file a lawsuit, and the other is to repeat the entire process all over again—not an appealing prospect, but it just might work.

Just a few loose ends to tie up before ending this section on Social Security: Don't put off applying. The date you file is very important. Your retroactive disability benefits only date back a maximum of one year before your filing date, regardless of how long you have been disabled. If you are too ill to apply in person, an application can be sent to you in the mail, or you may appoint a close friend or family member to be your representative. My parents spent many hours at the Social Security office helping me obtain my benefits.

If you are awarded benefits, you will also be eligible for Medicare, which is a very reasonable health insurance plan for the disabled and elderly. It pays 80 percent of approved doctors' fees. You are not eligible, however, until two years after you first become disabled and one year after your filing date.

SSI

For those of you who are disabled but have not worked long enough to be eligible for disability benefits, or for those of you who are eligible for benefits but whose monthly payments are not enough to keep you above the federally mandated poverty level, there is a program available to help. It is called Supplemental Security Income (SSI), a form of welfare that is administered through Social Security. Age is not a factor for this program; children as well as adults are eligible as long as their income is low. Since welfare programs are partially financed by the states, each state has its own rules and regulations.

Applying for SSI is similar to applying for disability benefits. If you can prove you are disabled and your income and your assets are within the guidelines, then you are eligible for SSI. Your income is the amount of money you receive each month from any source, such as disability benefits, stock dividends, money from friends and relatives, and so on. Also sometimes counted as income are things you receive in place of money, such as food and shelter. (Children living at home and not paying for food and housing will have some of their parents' assets and income counted against them.) Assets are things you own, such as stocks, bonds, savings and checking accounts, real estate, and some personal property. Your home is not counted as an asset. Your automobile as well as some personal possessions, depending on their value, may not be counted either. Social Security will inform you what is considered an asset and what is not.

If you think you might be eligible for SSI, it is easiest to apply for it at the same time you apply for disability benefits. You will be asked to fill out many forms and answer many questions. Bring with you proof of your income and assets, such as payroll stubs, insurance policies, bankbooks, and checking account statements. Once it is determined you are disabled and eligible for disability benefits, Social Security will compute your monthly earnings to see if you are eligible for SSI as well. SSI payments are typically much less than disability payments, and the amount differs from state to state. But the benefits are worth it if your disability benefits are not very high, or if you are disabled but have not worked enough to be eligible for Social Security disability.

MEDICAID

In addition to monthly checks, SSI recipients are eligible to receive Medicaid, a free health insurance plan for people with low income. Medicaid is also available to people with other sources of income, so long as that income is low enough to qualify. Medicaid pays 100 percent of approved doctors' fees. Unfortunately, Medicaid typically does not approve the total amount that most doctors charge so some doctors will not treat Medicaid patients. You may have to shop around a little to find a doctor who will.

HOUSING ASSISTANCE

SSI recipients and others with low income may also be eligible for rental subsidy programs. The state, county, or even some townships may have housing subsidy programs for the elderly, disabled, and low-income families. Some programs have low-rent housing units available. Others, such as the Section 8 rental subsidy program, may require you to find your own apartment. With either type of program, you are responsible for paying only 30 percent of your income in rent; the government pays the remainder. You should contact your local Social Security office, county welfare agency, or hospital social worker to see if there are any programs available in your area.

Applying for rental subsidy is the same as applying for any government program—more forms and more questions. When applying, bring all your Social Security records proving your disability and any financial information you have. As with SSI, these programs are dependent on your income and assets.

FOOD STAMPS

SSI recipients and others with low income may also be eligible for food stamps. As with rental subsidy, you usually apply for food stamps at a different agency than Social Security. But Social Security can inform you where that agency is located. Again, you will have lots of forms and lots of questions. And as with any of these programs, eligibility is dependent on your income and your assets. If you are eligible for food stamps, you are sent a certificate every month. You take this certificate with your identification card to a bank, where it is redeemed for the food stamps. (Actually, "stamps" is a misnomer. What you receive is a booklet filled with coupons of different denominations.) You then use these stamps at the grocery store the same way you would use cash. However, food stamps cannot be used for all grocery items, only for food products.

PERIODIC REVIEW

Once you've been approved for any of the above programs, including disability benefits, you are subject to periodic review. It may be done as frequently as once each year, or it might not happen for three or four years, but eventually Social Security and the other agencies will get around to reviewing your case. This process is typically the same as when you first applied. For disability benefits, you will need medical evidence and strong doctors' letters to prove that you are still disabled. If you applied for SSI or any welfare programs, you will have to prove that your income and assets have not changed substantially.

If your benefits are discontinued as a result of a review, you can request a hearing for reconsideration. This basically follows the same procedure as when you first applied. For disability, your case will be reviewed by an administrative law judge. Don't be discouraged if you have to go through this process. If you are truly disabled or needy, you have a very good chance of having your benefits reinstated.

In closing, please remember that there is financial help available, and for many of you, it would be worth your while to make the effort to obtain it. Disability benefits and other forms of assistance give you options, and options make coping with this illness a whole lot easier.

8

Advice for
Family and Friends

If it is true that every dark cloud has a silver lining, the silver lining of my illness would be this: It has enabled me to understand the many trials a whole family suffers when one of their own is hurting. For illness does not affect only the person it infects. The problems caused by chronic fatigue syndrome can splinter even the closest of relationships, which is why I felt it important to include this chapter for family and friends.

Caring for someone who is chronically ill is a labor of love. It is a labor because it is an arduous struggle with a disease whose demands are not limited to weeks, but to years. But the harshness of this labor is tempered by the mellifluence of love. The endeavor shines forth as a wonderful example of love's purest form: self-sacrifice.

Where do we find the strength to give so completely of ourselves? There is no genetic trait passed down over the generations that predisposes some to achieving this most noble of goals and others to failure. If it were as automatic as that, we would not esteem self-sacrificial love so highly. Selflessness is valued because it must be striven for.

Hardships require of us our excellence, but what is required is not beyond our grasp. If truth be told, none of us would choose to endure hardships of any kind, especially the hardships associated with illness. Choosing which is our portion to suffer, however, is a luxury we rarely enjoy. In this regard, loving and caring for someone who is chronically ill is the same as being chronically ill—you have no choice but to endure. Like ships foundering in a sudden storm, we brave the gales not because we want to, but because we have to. Often our finest moments are born not out of desire, but out of necessity.

Though I am chronically ill, I also know the pain of loving someone who is chronically ill. Countless times I would gladly have taken upon myself the pain of Shawn's illness— not solely for altruistic reasons, as many would suppose, but because to relieve her pain would relieve my own: Watching Shawn suffer hurt me more than words can express. Though my defenses could withstand the raging fury of my own illness, they were helpless against even the slightest whisper of Shawn's.

I am sure that for many of you, the pain of loving someone but being unable to effect his cure may seem almost unbearable. Through years of weaving close personal relationships, a fabric of concern entwines people with those who love them. If you are a spouse, parent, child, or friend of someone with CFS, many of your hopes and aspirations may be inextricably intertwined with those of your loved ones. When their dreams are shattered, so are yours.

The responsibility of caring for someone with CFS may have been placed squarely on your shoulders. Initially, you may have accepted this burden willingly, but have now found it difficult to bear as the months stretch into years. Sacrifices are easier to start than to sustain. If your loved one were acutely and temporarily ill, the challenge would not be as great. We would all prefer the satisfaction of being lifesavers to the prosaic endurance of being life-sustainers.

In contrast to the respect and admiration accorded those who care for the acutely ill, caring for the chronically ill is done in relative obscurity. This is because, to outsiders, there is nothing inspiring or triumphant about chronic illness. Everything associated with the term *chronic* has negative connotations. You never hear anyone claiming to be chronically happy or chronically in love. The only time you hear the word *chronic* is in relation to unceasing illness.

It is just that sense of endlessness, the inability to derive strength from knowing your trials will soon be over, that can make the future seem terribly discouraging. This is not just a temporary commitment; it demands a total readjustment of the family structure and responsibilities.

Resentment

Because of the continuous disruption this illness can cause in your lives, everyone in your family might harbor feelings of resentment at one time or another. This is quite understandable. The needs seem endless. No matter how much you do, it never seems to be enough. Feelings of frustration and irritability surface because you're overwhelmed by all that's required of you every day. Everything you planned for your lives may now seem hopelessly out of reach.

Countless problems and emotions must be dealt with each and every day. Your children may be having a hard time at school because they have a sibling or parent who is "different." You may even be losing some of your close friends because they don't understand this illness and are afraid it is contagious. Whatever the problem, it is important that you not neglect your own needs or the needs of the rest of your family. Everyone's emotional and physical strength must be kept up.

Because your loved one is at home sick, you may feel guilty when you spend time out enjoying yourself. You must remember, however, that your emotions need feeding as surely as your body does. Suppressing your own needs and feelings is unhealthy, and results in resentment, bitterness, and withdrawal.

Then you will be caring for your loved one not out of love, but because you feel it is your responsibility. This can't help but be perceived, and will create barriers as strong as any erected by this illness.

Don't Be Alone with Your Feelings

One of the most important pieces of advice I can give any friend or family member affected by CFS is to rely on the help of others. When our CFS support group first began, I imagined its sole purpose would be to help those of us with this illness cope with our affliction. I never dreamed it would also serve as a place where family and friends could find comfort and understanding.

It was wonderful to see their needs being met in ways we never envisioned. They were comforted by the realization that they were not alone, that there were others who understood the heartrending trials of caring for someone with CFS. You need to be honest about your feelings and share them with someone who cares, if not at a support group, then with a close friend or relative, or perhaps even a counselor. We all need support and understanding to cope with this traumatic illness. It is not a sign of weakness but a sign of strength to go to others for help.

Don't be afraid to include your loved one among the people you go to for help. When Shawn and I first became ill, I made the foolish mistake of keeping most of my emotions locked away, deep inside. I felt guilty burdening Shawn with them; it seemed selfish to ask her to help me. I hoped that if I ignored my feelings, the problems and resentments would just go away. Suppressed emotions don't go away; they fester and grow.

I have since learned the importance of being honest with Shawn. It does neither of us any good to hide our true feelings from each other. Relationships are based on sharing. They require trust, and trust is built on honesty. If problems are concealed, the sick person will come to feel isolated and unneeded. The two of you may drift apart. In the end you may have two people with resentments: the caregiver, trapped with pent-up emotions, and the patient, feeling untrustworthy and excluded from your life.

Of course, I try to be sensitive to Shawn's illness and not overwhelm her by expressing everything I am feeling at one time, but I don't deny my feelings in order to protect her. A balance must be achieved. If either of us is too ill to discuss something, we tell the other and save it for a day when we feel stronger.

Understanding Your Loved One's Needs

As you are no doubt aware, the changes wrought by CFS can make patients' lives feel painfully beyond their control. Discouragement comes easily when treatments don't work, and pangs of guilt are an all-too-common companion when patients realize the effect of their illness on family and friends. All the things that used to make life worth living—job, self-esteem, even simple pleasures—may no longer seem relevant. I make these points because it is important that you understand that chronically ill people have emotional, social, and spiritual needs, not just physical ones. You may be your loved one's only source of encouragement and support, so you need to be sensitive to all of these needs.

Preserving Independence

One emotional need common to people with CFS is the need to feel independent. When someone else does all their cooking and cleaning, perhaps even makes many of their decisions, it is easy for them to become dependent on other people and lose their identity as adults. Victims of CFS need to be treated as adults and not children. They should not be kept in the dark medically. Nothing should be hidden from them, because they will see right through it. Try not to be overprotective or smothering, and respect your loved one's privacy as well.

Family members should trust the judgment of their loved ones in regard to their limitations. People with CFS should never be pressured into activities they are not well enough to do. On the other hand, at times they may need to be active in order to keep their spirits up. Express your concerns, but then allow your loved one to make the decision without imposing guilt. People with CFS know their limitations.

You should also try to be supportive of any treatments that are undertaken. Even if you have reservations, your loved one must have the freedom to make the final decision.

Remember to think of the chronically ill as people and not patients. Be sensitive to their limitations, but don't define them by their illness. Your loved one is no less a person because of this disease. Many people with CFS feel useless and superfluous. They need to have family and friends share their lives with them, allowing them to feel accepted and attached. People with CFS still need to feel important, so continue to go to them for advice or help. This allows them the opportunity to contribute to the family. Your loved ones need to know that you value them, not just for what they do, but for who they are.

Acceptance and Understanding

Another very important emotional need is to feel accepted and understood. You can help with this by acknowledging the hurt your loved one is experiencing and by expressing your concern and support. Acknowledging pain is as simple as saying, "I am so sorry that you are hurting. It hurts me to see you struggling. I want you to know that I will always be here for you if you need me." Don't belittle your loved one's pain by giving pat answers like, "Don't worry, you'll be well soon," or "At least your illness isn't fatal." If you don't acknowledge the severity of this affliction, your loved one will feel isolated and alone. Learn to listen, not only to what is said, but to what is meant. Many people say they are okay but really mean they are hurting.

Unfortunately, I have met family members who have a snap-out-of-it mentality about chronic illness. They delude themselves into thinking they are offering support and encouragement when they push and prod their loved one to act healthy. In reality, they are doing nothing but venting their impatience and frustration on an innocent victim. Before we were married, Shawn lived with her mother in Michigan. Her mother bore the brunt of Shawn's depression and irritability, which are the hallmarks of this illness, as well as taking care of her daily physical and financial needs. Never once did she make Shawn feel guilty for being unable to be well. Her encouragement always took the form of, "It's all right that you're ill," rather than "I can't believe you're still ill."

Be Realistic—But Not Negative

Acknowledging pain is not the same as constantly dwelling on the illness, always emphasizing the negative. Be aware of what you say and how you treat someone with CFS. I have met families who continually say that their loved one's life is passing by, that his potential is being wasted. They constantly bring up the fact that their loved one is missing out on the best years of life and will never be able to relive them. This type of negative talk is not helpful.

The chronically ill measure their lives in months, not minutes. Healthy people run their lives by the clock: 45 minutes to get ready in the morning; 15-minute coffee break; 30 minutes for lunch; 25 minutes to drive home from work. If I thought of my life as minutes slipping by, I would not be able to cope with this illness another day.

My world is regulated not by the clock, but by the calendar. When I first became ill, I felt time rushing by faster than I could measure. Every day I was ill was a further postponement of my life. All my friends and relatives seemed to be passing me by.

It took me years to unlearn a healthy man's time reference, but I have finally succeeded. I no longer measure time from the beginning of my life, but from the end. I no longer look backward to see how many years have passed, but take hope by looking forward to how many years remain.

People with CFS already feel that in many ways they are waiting to live. They don't need to be constantly reminded of it. Without minimizing the illness, you should try to stress the positive. Try to make your loved one's life as normal and as enjoyable as possible.

Running Interference

Your loved one's social needs are also very important. But one thing that can stand in the way of social pleasure is the insensitive remarks of other people. This is a place where you, as a concerned friend or relative, can help by being a social go-between. Perhaps a few examples of the situations I've faced will show you what I mean.

I find it very discomforting to answer probing questions about my illness. It can make me feel like an oddity at a circus sideshow. I don't believe these people are trying purposely to be cruel. They just don't realize how much pain their insensitive questions can inflict.

Then there are the incredulous comments: "You look so well!" More often than not the sentiment is well intentioned, but those four little words never encourage me; they make me feel stupid. I never know what to reply. I usually say that I try hard to look well, hoping to convey the thought that I'm not the type who seeks to magnify his illness.

Incredibly, some people have actually told me they were envious of my life-style. They wished they could do nothing but sleep and eat all day! It takes every ounce of self-control I can muster not to fall on my knees right there and ask the Lord to grant their request.

Other people send subtle signals of impatience. They say they are sympathetic, but their underlying message is "Why don't you try harder to beat this thing?" They don't understand that living with this illness is like being precariously balanced on a rickety old raft, swept up in the middle of an emotional and physical maelstrom. They don't see how hard I fight every day with all of my strength just to keep afloat. If these people really understood my illness, they would marvel at how strong I truly am.

With insensitive people to deal with and bewildering situations to face, your loved one may begin to shy away from social situations. If you can run interference, helping people understand CFS and the way it affects your loved one, you will make it easier for him to be around them.

When people who are unfamiliar with CFS come to visit, it may be appropriate to take them aside and briefly explain the nature of the illness. Many people feel uncomfortable visiting the sick because they don't know what to say, or they may even feel guilty because they are well. You need to be the facilitator in awkward situations, trying to make everyone feel comfortable and at ease.

In addition to explaining the illness to others, you can also make the needs of your loved one known. People are often nice enough to offer their help, but when a need arises, it is not always easy to ask. You can let people know how they can help, financially, physically, or emotionally.

Offering Your Help

It is very difficult to need financial help and even more difficult to receive it. If you want to help financially, you should consider having your loved one's bills delivered to you rather than having him give them to you every month. This may alleviate some of the guilt involved and allow a greater sense of independence.

Aside from helping your loved one financially, you may also want to make a contribution to one of the CFS organizations listed in Appendix C, or to one of the many facilities doing research on CFS.

Being active in the political arena is another way you can help. More funding is needed for CFS research, and public and government awareness needs to be raised. This means that a lot of letters need to be written to senators and representatives. My parents have taken over this chore for us. They have given hundreds of photocopied letters to friends, relatives, and associates to send to Washington. Many of our other relatives and friends have distributed letters in other states and districts. The various CFS organizations can provide you with names and addresses to write to.

Keeping Up-to-Date

When you are very ill, it is not easy to keep up on all the pertinent information on CFS. Our family and friends keep their eyes and ears open for any possible treatments or information that might help. They read articles and maintain correspondence with support groups and doctors.

Another way to show your support is by attending support group meetings with your loved one. It is wise for any family member or close friend to attend at least one meeting because it will help you better understand the effects of CFS. Since Shawn and I often feel too ill to attend meetings, my parents attend for us. This ensures that we don't miss any new information.

Sharing the Burden

Another important way to help your loved one is by helping with his physical needs. But it is very difficult to ask for help from others because this illness persists for so many years. Maybe friends could alternate helping, one cooking a meal one week, another doing laundry, and so on. Coordinating all this help for your loved one is a valuable service, and you can even turn it into a social occasion (but you should remember that even short visits can be draining).

Our friends and family know that our physical limitations make it very difficult to socialize. We find it draining to go out or to entertain. They overcome this by occasionally bringing a sub sandwich or a pizza, sharing a meal and some time with us.

Don't Forget the Little Things

There are so many little but meaningful things you can do to encourage and support someone who is ill. In fact, your imagination is the only limitation to the ways you can lend your support. You could give flowers, records, books, bubble bath, favorite foods, cable TV, and crafts. If your loved one is too ill to read, perhaps you could read a special book into a tape recorder.

Even a card or a phone call can give the encouragement needed to endure. When Shawn was too ill to leave the house or have anyone visit, mail was the highlight of her day. She desperately needed to know that other people cared. You can't imagine how intense this need is for people who are chronically ill. Some people who had never even met us sent us cards, letting us know they were praying for us. To know that someone cared enough to pray for us always touched us deeply. Touch is also an important way of expressing your love and concern, especially when your loved one is feeling isolated and alone.

While it is important to do everything you can to be supportive of your loved one, it is just as important that you not neglect the other members of the family. Be sensitive to the way they are affected by this illness. They will be facing their own problems as well, and they should not be made to feel as if their struggles are unimportant. Their problems may not be as devastating as CFS is, but they are still painful and need to be acknowledged. And even though you are hurting for your loved one, it is important to allow other family members to be happy. They are growing and moving on; rejoice with them.

CFS is very demanding. Each one of you must learn how to live with this devastating affliction. With everything you do and with everything you say, try to imagine what it would be like to be in your loved one's position. If whatever you say or do is based in love, more than likely it will be received with gratitude and affection. My prayer for you is that, through this trial, your relationships will grow even closer.

9

Questions
and Answers

A n interview with **James M. Oleske, M.D., M.P.H.,** Professor in the Department of Pediatrics at the University of Medicine and Dentistry, New Jersey Medical School; and Director of the Division of Allergy, Immunology, and Infectious Diseases.

Over the years, this syndrome has been referred to by many different names. What are some of the other names for chronic fatigue syndrome?

This syndrome has been referred to as chronic Epstein-Barr virus (CEBV), chronic mononucleosis, epidemic and sporadic neuromyasthenia, myalgic encephalomyelitis, postviral fatigue syndrome, neurasthenia, Icelandic disease, and others.

Is chronic fatigue syndrome contagious?

Among individuals who have the sporadic form of this infection, there does not seem to be an epidemic strain of virus that causes CFS; otherwise we would see whole families coming down with the syndrome. When we do see more than one family member, it is somewhat unusual.

If Epstein-Barr virus is involved, then the people who are initially infected with the virus go through a short phase when they excrete large amounts of the virus in their saliva. At this time, they may be considered more infectious and contagious than individuals who are not in such a state. However, Epstein-Barr virus, like all herpesviruses, causes lifelong latent infection with various periods of reactivation and spontaneous excretion of the virus, regardless of whether the individual is symptomatic or not. From present evidence, it does not appear that the patient with CFS is at higher risk of transmitting the disease than an asymptomatic individual. Therefore, even if the EB virus is involved, it is the virus that is contagious whereas the syndrome does not appear to be. And since 90 percent of the adult population has already been exposed to the EB virus, it is not an infection that most people need to be concerned about.

However, it may be that other cofactors, in particular another virus, are related to this syndrome. A newly identified herpesvirus, known as human herpesvirus 6, is being examined as a possible agent that could cause CFS. If another new viral agent were discovered, then we would have to reevaluate the possibility of person-to-person spread of infectious CFS. But, for the present time, most of the CFS cases are not contagious and do not appear to be an epidemic strain.

There is a form of CFS that appears to occur in epidemics. The most recent example of this is the outbreak, as defined by Dr. Cheney, in the Lake Tahoe region. In this setting, there appeared to be more rapid person-to-person spread, but with a shorter period of symptomatology. This may, in fact, be a different variant of this disease process. In this situation, there appears to be some increased contagion as well as an increase in the ability of the same type of syndrome to be transmitted from one adult individual to another.

As time goes by, do people with CFS tend to get better, get worse, or stay the same?

I think that one of the problems for individuals who have this syndrome is that it's difficult to judge day by day whether they are getting better or worse. In my experience, over long periods of time—and I'm talking about sometimes five to ten years—individuals seem to slowly get better. Usually when they look back and ask, "Do I feel better than I did, say, a year ago?" the answer is yes. It is hard to judge progress in terms of days because a patient experiences peaks and valleys for days at a time, but overall, there is a slow progression upward. So, there is quite a bit of fluctuation in the symptoms but, I think, a gradual improvement. Sometimes to the patient it is an imperceptible, gradual improvement, but a gradual improvement overall. My general impression is that most people with this syndrome do feel better after long periods of time.

Are people with CFS more susceptible to other infections?

Yes and no. Most patients are not at risk of developing serious infections, but there are other patients who are susceptible to lesser viral infections. There is certainly a group of patients that we have seen, about one-third to one-half, who have low antibody levels and seem to be more susceptible to allergic-like diseases. In my opinion, because of their antibody deficiency, they are more likely to be susceptible to other viral infections, especially in their weakened condition from CFS. This is one of the reasons that our staff, in particular, has suggested the use of intravenous gamma globulin.

Should people with CFS donate blood?

Any patient with a chronic infection should not donate blood. I have seen CFS patients with some anemia. The disease itself, and their own requirements for strength and rest, would dictate that they should not donate blood. It is possible that they may be more infectious to other people by donating blood, but that's not the issue. The issue, more importantly, is that donating blood is not recommended for anybody with the kind of chronic symptomatology, weakness, and fatigue that a patient with this syndrome has.

Should women with CFS be concerned about becoming pregnant?

The data based upon women who have had the syndrome and who have had children indicate that there are no demonstrable deforming effects to the fetus and that the women have been able to have healthy and normal children. Obviously, physicians are always concerned about recommending pregnancy to anybody who is on long-term medication or who has a chronic disease. If a woman with CFS does become pregnant, any medication she is taking needs to be evaluated in light of the pregnancy.

Also, the stress of pregnancy may worsen this fatiguelike syndrome. Paradoxically, it may even make it better. We don't understand how this syndrome works or how pregnancy affects it. In general, pregnancy is associated with an impaired immune response in the pregnant woman, which allows her to carry the fetus. Because of this, I certainly wouldn't wholeheartedly recommend that women who have CFS become pregnant, for their own sake. But all the present evidence shows that they can have normal babies and that there is no increased risk.

Should people with CFS avoid vaccines for other illnesses, such as the flu or polio, and is there any difference between live and dead vaccines?

I think that any of the killed viral vaccines, like the flu vaccines, are certainly recommended and may be helpful for someone with a chronic illness. There is some cause for concern about live vaccines, such as polio. Since most CFS patients are adults and polio is not usually one of their recommended vaccines, I would avoid live polio vaccines. I would also avoid measles, mumps, and rubella vaccines, but I would encourage the flu vaccine.

Is there any special information CFS patients need to know in case they are hospitalized?

Only that I feel it's important that every patient with CFS have a primary care physician who is at least sympathetic to their problem and understanding of their disease process. One of the problems that I have noted in my involvement with CFS patients is the lack of doctors who are willing to be responsive to their needs. CFS patients cannot continually rely on the resources of the immunologist or infectious disease specialist to provide primary care.

I myself find that I am overwhelmed and unable to respond to the case after case, document after document, that needs to be filled out for Social Security, or what have you, and also provide ongoing day-in and day-out care for the multiple complaints someone with this chronic syndrome has. It's imperative that the pool of physicians who are willing to take care of CFS patients be built up. And particularly, these physicians should be primary care specialists, like GPs, family practitioners, or internists. I don't think that primary care can be rendered by the subspecialist because he or she just does not do a good job.

Is there anything an emergency room doctor would need to know about CFS?

Every patient with a chronic illness should have a physician who knows the syndrome and who can talk to the emergency doctor.

In particular, I think there is no general worry about penicillin allergy or drug allergy. The physician in the emergency room should be informed that the patient has a chronic fatiguelike syndrome. And he should certainly consult the caring physician, whether it's a primary physician or, in an emergency, the subspecialist.

What criteria do you use when making a diagnosis of CFS?

There are some general guidelines. The patient should be ill for at least six months, fatigue should be a prominent symptom, and the individual should be somewhat disabled by this illness.

There are also other associated multiple findings that we see with this syndrome, especially related to the central nervous system. These include fatigue, sleep disturbances, inappropriate thought patterns, inability to concentrate, a lot of nonspecific complaints related to nausea or vomiting, abdominal cramping, muscle pain, muscle cramping, and joint pains and aches. The classical findings of fatigue, apparent central nervous system involvement, and duration of symptoms for longer than six months are very important.

Laboratory confirmatory data vary. We used to like to see elevated EBV titers, especially elevated early antigen (EA) titers and depressed levels of EB nuclear antigen (EBNA) titers, but that no longer seems to be diagnostically significant. Our particular staff has been so impressed with low immunoglobulin (antibody) levels, in particular immunoglobulin G (IgG) subclass deficiency, that we test subclass levels routinely. When we find a deficiency, that helps us to firm up the diagnosis.

Probably more important than anything else, however, is that the patient with CFS, or suspected CFS, deserves to have a full workup done in order to rule out other illnesses that may mask themselves and be more treatable than CFS. This is why I can't emphasize enough the importance of having a good internist, family physician, or primary care specialist involved with the subspecialist who's concerned more with CFS. The disservice often done to the patient is not diagnosing lupus when it's present, or lymphoma, or some other disease process and just saying it's chronic fatigue syndrome.

Will the standard diagnostic tests, such as urinalysis or common blood tests, reveal anything significant for CFS patients?

Usually not. The most important thing to emphasize is that the physician evaluating and caring for the patient with CFS should not miss any treatable condition. Therefore, standard diagnostic tests should be performed during the initial evaluation and should be redone periodically to test for other diseases that could be associated with CFS.

Obviously, when a patient develops a new sign, symptom, or abnormality, it shouldn't be written off as just CFS. Therefore, I think that it is important to have periodic health evaluations every year or two. And part of the health evaluation is routine diagnostic tests, such as blood tests or urinalysis. These tests don't specifically help in the diagnosis of CFS, but they should be a part of any physician's routine health examination. If something abnormal is found in those tests, I hope that the physician wouldn't write it off simply as CFS. He should always make sure that there isn't anything else wrong.

Is the monospot blood test, used for diagnosing infectious mononucleosis, useful in diagnosing CFS?

No, the simple monospot test is really not useful. In fact, even the more specific EBV titer test is no longer considered diagnostic. In the beginning, when we started treating patients, there was some hope that a drop in titers or a change from early antigen (EA) to Epstein-Barr nuclear antigen (EBNA) might signal an improvement in symptoms. But that is no longer the case. I have not seen in my patients any variation of symptomatology definitely correlated with EBV titers. Healthy individuals can have similar EBV titers to CFS patients, so we no longer rely on these tests to make a diagnosis. With time, when we become better able to specifically diagnose this syndrome, we will have better tests that will indicate whether an individual does or does not have this syndrome. Hopefully, these tests will also allow us to evaluate a change in the severity of symptoms.

How do you distinguish between mononucleosis and CFS?

Mononucleosis and CFS have many common features, such as fatigue, but many are quite different. Patients with CFS generally do not have substantial enlargement of the lymph nodes, but rather intermittent node tenderness. They tend not to run high fevers, but may be feverish. They do not generally have an enlarged liver or spleen, major changes in blood count profiles, or hypersensitivity to ampicillin as do patients with mononucleosis.

When someone's symptoms persist for longer than six months, and there is little tonsilar pharyngitis, then I'm more likely to call an illness chronic fatigue syndrome as opposed to acute mono. Remember, acute mono can be a devastating disease, present sometimes for three or four months or even a year.

Some patients have low or absent EBNA on their EBV serology blood tests. What is the significance of this?

This is one area where EBV titer tests are significant. EBNA is the antibody that normally rises in someone who is recovering from an EBV infection over a long time. So the presence of rising titers to EBNA may herald the onset of recovery, although this isn't clear-cut. There is an awful lot of fluctuation in EBV titers within individual patients. I think it's fair to say that if someone had persistently rising EBNA titers and was improving, that is consistent with what we see happening in individuals who recover from an EBV infection.

The significance of negative EBNA is that the body is having a problem mounting an effective immune response. Most CFS patients have positive EBNA titers, but about 20 percent don't. These people are not experiencing the normal immune response.

What is the connection between allergy and CFS?

It appears that patients with CFS are more likely than the general population to have allergies uncovered during the course of their illness. I think this is linked somewhat to our observation of abnormalities in immune responses, especially in the subclasses of IgG. It appears that it's possible, and likely, that this syndrome is able to affect normal immune functions to the point where, if you will, allergies are unmasked in an individual who otherwise would not suffer from allergies—just as subclass deficiencies may develop in individuals who may otherwise not have those.

Now, it may be just the opposite—it's the old argument of which came first, the chicken or the egg. I guess it's possible to argue that people with allergies or people with subclass deficiencies are predisposed to developing CFS. Until we do long prospective studies—studies that follow a group of patients over a long period of time and compare their data with other groups—we'll never really be able to answer that question.

Can allergies make CFS symptoms worse?

No question, and the one thing that a physician can do is make life better for CFS patients by seeing to it that their various treatable symptoms are treated. Though we may not be able to do anything about the fatigue, if an individual with CFS does suffer from allergies, simple treatment of allergic symptoms may help.

Medications that don't cause further fatigue should be used. For example, the use of Seldane, an antihistamine that doesn't cross the blood-brain barrier, versus an antihistamine that would make someone more sleepy, makes eminent sense. In fact, several of my CFS patients who had persistent allergy symptoms improved with the use of Seldane and other types of antihistamines, although their CFS did not go away. And I think the job of the physician is to try to help the patient feel better.

What about allergy shots and allergy desensitization?

I have no direct experience with whether allergy shots would help someone with CFS. Certainly, if someone has severe inhalant allergies that can be documented by skin tests, a cautious course of immunotherapy wouldn't be out of the question.

Should people with CFS avoid things they are allergic to, such as pets?

This is probably a good point. I think that animal dander and dust exposure should be kept to a minimum for patients with CFS. You have to weigh this, however, against the psychological benefit of pets. Sometimes individuals who are severely bedridden benefit substantially from the companionship of pets. So anything you do obviously has to be weighed against which benefits you the most. But for individuals who don't have a strong affinity for having a pet, I would recommend against having pets if they are allergic to animals.

Do patients' symptoms become worse during certain allergy seasons?

I'm not sure it's their symptoms of CFS that get worse, but when they have an exacerbation of their allergies, they feel miserable. It is sometimes difficult to separate when they're having an exacerbation of their CFS from when they're just having a miserable exacerbation of their allergies.

Is there any evidence that CFS affects one sex or race more than another?

The male-to-female ratio is fairly consistent throughout the United States, with a 2:1 or 3:1 female predominance. The racial ratio is much more predominantly white, and I don't know if we have a clear understanding whether this is purely racial origin or is perhaps related to social and economic factors. The predominance of Caucasians who seem to suffer from this syndrome is striking, however.

Is there any evidence of a family link or a genetic predisposition toward CFS?

The finding of IgG subclass deficiencies in some of our patients may indicate some genetic linkage. At the present time, we have a few cases in which mothers and daughters in particular are both infected with this syndrome. But these are unusual cases. We don't yet have an answer to this question, and again, this is one of many problems that require long prospective studies.

If someone is going to have a serious complication from this infection, is it more likely to occur at the onset of the illness?

In my experience, I have not seen complications of CFS occurring after three or four years. I think people are miserable and tired, and slowly get better, but I don't see a period when they are any more susceptible to complications.

What are the possible serious complications associated with CFS?

There are few medical complications that affect patients with CFS. My impression is that most of the complications are psychological, and job and school related—patients being so fatigued that their normal life-styles are interrupted. There are some medical problems, such as joint pain, abdominal pain, and headaches, that can be very severe. In general, however, there has been no permanent damage due to CFS-associated complications, outside of the fact that they further add to the misery of this disease.

I have not noticed any severe complications in my patients or been impressed with any that have been noted in the medical literature. I have not observed any higher incidence of malignancies, heart disease, permanent liver disease, or any organ failure induced by CFS. In other words, CFS is not a degenerative disease, and I don't see patients developing renal or heart failure.

What is encephalitis, and how does it relate to CFS?

The general term *encephalopathy* means "inflammation of the brain." This results from a variety of different things. Direct infection of the brain by a virus, we tend to call encephalitis. The virus causes changes in the brain, causing many different symptoms similar to those experienced by patients with CFS. Inflammation of the brain can also be induced by a variety of other causes, such as drugs or heavy metals, like lead.

Postinfectious encephalitis is the inflammation of the brain in reaction to a virus that was previously present.

It may be in CFS that there is direct infection of the central nervous system, including the brain, by one or more viruses. Or it may be that the symptoms that we see in CFS, which seem to suggest some type of central nervous system involvement, may be a postinfectious encephalopathy.

Is there any link between CFS and arthritis?

There is a definite link in the medical literature between severe mononucleosis caused by Epstein-Barr virus and the possible unmasking of juvenile rheumatoid arthritis (JRA) in children. Some people feel that severe mono in a child may be linked to genetic susceptibility to JRA. If EBV is involved in CFS, then there may be a connection.

I've been impressed in my patients with CFS that a number of them, possibly one-third, have joint symptoms, arthralgias, and aches and pains. This probably is not related to a collagen vascular disease like rheumatoid arthritis, but clearly it may reflect changes in the body induced by chronic fatigue syndrome.

Do people with CFS need to be concerned about developing arthritis?

I don't think they'll develop severe crippling arthritis, the worrisome type. But one-third of them will have joint pains and muscle aches.

Is cancer a disease that people with CFS need to be concerned with?

At the present time, we have no evidence to suggest that this is a problem. If the EB virus is involved somehow, we know that it is linked to the genetic predisposition for Burkitt's lymphoma, which is a cancer found mainly among blacks from Africa; and nasopharyngeal carcinoma, which occurs predominantly in Orientals. We have not seen such a linkage to a malignancy in Caucasians, and Caucasians are the most likely to get CFS. Even if EBV is involved, we haven't seen lymphomas in CFS patients. So the answer so far is no; there is no definite implicated cancer in patients with CFS.

Epstein-Barr virus is often associated with AIDS. Should people with CFS be afraid of AIDS?

The patient with CFS is a member of society as a whole and should be as afraid of developing AIDS as any other member of society. However, AIDS is spread by very specific methods—sexual contact, IV drug abuse and from infected mother to unborn child. If a CFS patient is sexually promiscuous, is gay, or is an IV drug abuser, then he has just as much risk of developing AIDS as anybody else. And if he does get AIDS, he probably will have a worse problem with it because he's already debilitated and may be infected with one of the infectious agents that appear to make AIDS worse.

However, patients with CFS are no more likely to get AIDS than anybody else if they don't take part in those risk factors that are known to spread AIDS. EBV is not the virus that causes AIDS; it's just an opportunistic infection that affects AIDS patients. If the EB virus is involved with CFS, then someone with CFS who got AIDS would just be an individual who happened to have one of the opportunistic infections carried—and would be that much the worse for it.

Should CFS patients be concerned about using blood products, such as gamma globulin or transfer factor?

We have very clear evidence that the AIDS virus is not transmitted by gamma globulin. Because of the studies done on how gamma globulin is processed, with the removal of any possible virus during this process, I can comfortably state that gamma globulin is safe, especially from the AIDS virus.

The same cannot be said for transfer factor. There are no cases I know of where AIDS was transferred by transfer factor; however, enough studies have not been done. It is not clearly known if the storing and freeze-drying process that goes into making transfer factor would deactivate the AIDS virus. It would seem unlikely that a viral agent would survive the production of transfer factor from lymphocytes, but there is potential. And since, to my knowledge, appropriate studies have not been done, we cannot make the same claims about the safety of transfer factor as we would about gamma globulin.

If transfer factor is made from a single individual who does not have any evidence of AIDS, then obviously it would be safe to use that kind of product. However, when transfer factor is made from many individuals and those individuals have not been screened for AIDS, then there would be some risk involved.

Should the general population be afraid of getting CFS through blood products?

No. There is no evidence whatsoever that there is any danger to the general population of coming down with CFS through the use of blood and blood products.

Can you explain the significance of the discovery of the human herpesvirus 6?

HHV6 is a unique herpesvirus that may be either the prime cause or a cofactor in the development of CFS. Dr. Gallo's lab at the National Institutes of Health has demonstrated this virus, but studies so far have not linked it directly to CFS. The discovery of this virus may be a major breakthrough. It may very well be that to get CFS, you need to have both EB virus infection and this new virus. It is also possible that infection with this new virus is the sole cause of CFS or that the virus causes other, as yet unrecognized diseases, but not CFS.

Can you describe what happened in the 1984–85 CFS outbreak in Lake Tahoe, Nevada?

It appears that in Lake Tahoe, as opposed to a good number of patients I have seen, as well as those described by Dr. Straus and Dr. Jones, there was an *epidemic* of a CFS-like illness. This occurred over a shorter period of time as well as over a closed population, with more rapid clearing of symptoms spontaneously. There also seemed to possibly be more direct neurological involvement, as demonstrated by positive NMR scans, that we have not seen in our nonepidemic CFS patients.

The Tahoe outbreak peaked in 1985, and the incidence of new cases has declined. Twenty percent of the patients have somewhat recovered. Whether it is the same process or a different one, we're not sure. Obviously, it's very important to study the epidemic and nonepidemic cases of CFS.

In your opinion, how serious an illness is CFS?

There are a number of individuals with this syndrome who are completely disabled. There are others who have varying degrees of disability. One of our difficulties is the lack of prospective studies to look at this problem. It's clear that it will take a national organization like the Centers for Disease Control to really come to grips with the scope of the problem, as they did for AIDS.

Generally speaking, what is your opinion of possible treatments with harmful side effects, such as interferon, or treatments that are not federally approved, such as Isoprinosine?

Any patient with CFS, or any chronic illness, runs the risk of being desperate enough to seek therapies that may be questionable. In the long run, an individual with a chronic illness is less harmed if he has a legitimate physician who understands this syndrome and is willing to provide advice on safe and effective therapies. There is no question that there may be a magic answer out there, but for every possible magic answer, there may be many tragedies lurking for an individual with CFS.

It is clear that the goal of CFS treatment should be controlling the expression of the infection. This may take a combination of antiviral medications and medications which manipulate the immune system. Random guessing with treatments of interferon, transfer factor, or Isoprinosine, in an uncontrolled fashion, will never give the correct answers.

It is important that appropriate studies be well funded that will rapidly look at the available treatments and determine which ones are most likely to help the vast majority of patients with CFS. Unfortunately, as difficult as it is for a CFS patient to accept, the only real way of getting answers is through controlled testing. And until we start doing those tests in a rapid fashion, the patient with CFS runs the risk of trying medications that may not help him and, worse yet, may cause harm.

Generally speaking, what is your advice to patients suffering with CFS?

People with CFS should try to optimize the goals they have. They should concentrate on what is important to them and not push themselves to accomplish everything. For example, if someone is in college, he should try to finish college if he can and not worry about having three jobs and working out. If someone has a job, he should concentrate on the job and not his aerobics class. They're going to have to give up things. They're going to have to rest. They're going to have to slowly recover from this fatigue syndrome over a period of years.

There are a number of simple symptomatic therapies, depending on how ill the patient is. Obviously, if the patient is able to function and lead a relatively normal life, then we try not to interfere. The therapies we try depend on how severe the symptoms are.

For patients with many joint pains, and aches and pains, a nonsteroidal anti-inflammatory may be helpful. For patients with tremendous central nervous system involvement, such as head-aches or thinking problems, we've toyed with the use of Diamox. It is a diuretic which may possibly lower central nervous system pressure. Sinequan, an antidepressant, seems to help relieve the fatigue associated with CFS, not just by its antidepressant effect but by some unknown effect. When patients have low antibody or IgG subclass deficiency, treatment with gamma globulin may help.

It seems that the antiviral drugs available, such as acyclovir, haven't been of benefit in these patients. Obviously, other immunostimulants, like transfer factor or Isoprinosine, need to be evaluated in appropriate controlled studies. Answers need to be derived so we can help patients with this syndrome. In the meantime, some of these medications may help.

Also, it is helpful just having a physician following a patient, making sure that a new symptom that develops is not a harbin-ger of another illness that can be treated with some other medications. This prevents someone from ignoring a cough just because they were told they have CFS, when that cough could possibly be pneumonia. It is very important to have a caring physician who is willing to evaluate and respond to the needs of the patient, so every symptom that develops is not just automati-cally written off as CFS. It's also important for the patient with

CFS and his physician to try to avoid desperate attempts at therapies with possibly dangerous medications.

Can you briefly explain your research efforts using gamma globulin as a possible treatment for CFS and specifically explain your use of the IgG subclass blood test?

The major reason we began using IV gamma globulin was that, as an immunologist, I had already used lots of IV gamma globulin in patients who have antibody deficiencies. When we began seeing CFS patients in 1981, it was striking that when we tested the total immunoglobulin levels, they were in the low normal range. This was surprising because these people had experienced multiple infections in the past. When we looked further, however, and broke down the IgG into its subclasses, it became apparent that one-third to one-half of our patients had depressed subclass levels of immunoglobulin (antibodies). This, combined with the observation that they had recurrent fevers, sometimes indicative of infection, led us to try trials of IV gamma globulin on those patients with subclass deficiency.

In the initial group of patients seen, we saw 70 percent clinical improvement in symptoms. Based on that data, we did turn to the companies that make gamma globulin. Along with Dr. James Jones of National Jewish Hospital in Colorado, we have tried to encourage its use and have written protocols for controlled studies to evaluate gamma globulin and its role in treating CFS. Unfortunately, so far those controlled studies have not been supported. It is difficult for a busy clinical service to support doing controlled studies without the financial backing of the companies who make the products. We're hopeful that these studies will be undertaken.

I think it's clear that gamma globulin may be, like nonsteroidal anti-inflammatories and other medications, helpful in relieving some of the symptoms suffered by patients with CFS. Again, the goal should always be to make the patient feel better.

So you have found that, even though the overall tests for immune deficiency may be normal, when you go further and break down the IgG into subclasses, a significant number of CFS patients have abnormal subclass levels?

Yes, and this is the group that would most likely benefit from IV gamma globulin.

What do you see as the future of CFS; what can patients look forward to?

There is now interest in this illness by the Centers for Disease Control in Atlanta and the National Institutes of Health in Bethesda. This disease is no longer considered a myth disease, and patients with this syndrome are not considered malingerers. In fact, there is a real solid group of patients with a chronic fatigue syndrome that seems to be related to viral infections; whether it's Epstein-Barr virus, HHV6, or some other virus, time will tell.

I think there is going to be rapid development in the area of more specific diagnostic tests. This testing must be developed because there are many people who consider themselves as having CFS who don't. In fact, they may have other treatable diseases, either organic or psychological. And unfortunately, there are many skeptical physicians because they cannot pin down a diagnosis.

One of the best hopes is to develop a single test or a series of tests that allow us to make a more firm diagnosis of CFS. However, once we get that diagnostic test and are more secure in our knowledge of the cause of this disease, we will be able to become more rational in how we approach this disease from a therapeutic standpoint.

10
___
Research
Perspectives

___

By **Stephen E. Straus, M.D.,** head of the Medical Virology Section, Laboratory of Clinical Investigation/National Institute of Allergy and Infectious Diseases, and National Institutes of Health, and **Janet Dale, R.N.,** research coordinator of the Medical Virology Section, Laboratory of Clinical Investigation/National Institute of Allergy and Infectious Diseases, National Institutes of Health.

What is the illness about which Gregg Fisher feels compelled to write? Its associated symptoms are characteristic of many diseases and thereby lack identity as a unique disorder. The Centers for Disease Control has suggested a uniform case definition for research purposes, but there is still no diagnostic marker, or acceptable hypothesis of causation. The prognosis is uncertain and there is no cure. And, if these factors weren't enough of a frustration, many doubt the existence of this illness.

Many people explain this illness in terms of the properties and behavior of the Epstein-Barr virus. Unfortunately, it is by no means certain that they are focusing on the proper villain.

While it may be preferable for the one who suffers to identify some culprit rather than to be devoid of any rational explanation for his misery, we as research scientists must be more critical.

Today, in 1988, the Epstein-Barr virus must be viewed as one possible cause of illnesses like Gregg's. The notion that Epstein-Barr virus can lead to an illness with chronic fatigue has evolved since 1982, when it was first formally proposed by Martin Tobi and his colleagues in Israel. Their initial observation was that individuals with persisting fatigue and recurrent sore throat, tender lymph glands, and a variety of other problems possess unusual profiles of antibodies to Epstein-Barr virus proteins. Additionally, their symptoms resembled patterns that accompany Epstein-Barr virus–induced infectious mononucleosis; thus, it was reasoned that the chronic illness represents the manifestations of persistent infection with that virus.

By 1985, further studies confirmed Tobi's observation and noted that a variety of subtle immunologic abnormalities could also be detected in many patients. The abnormalities were of a type not seen or expected in acute Epstein-Barr virus infection, and suggested that perhaps an immune abnormality is the predominant problem in lieu of a specific infection.

Two additional observations made between 1985 and 1987 have strengthened this alternative hypothesis. First, it was shown that healthy people can have antibody profiles similar to those of some patients with the chronic fatigue syndrome. Specifically, antibodies to Epstein-Barr virus early antigens can persist at low levels for a few years after acute Epstein-Barr virus–induced infectious mononucleosis. Thus, antibodies to the viral early antigens are not diagnostic indicators of disease. Second, the types of symptoms reported by patients with the chronic fatigue syndrome were noted to be quite common, to follow a variety of different types of infections, or at times to begin insidiously rather than being heralded by an infectious illness.

The research findings of the past few years have not dealt a death blow to the hypothesis that EBV can lead to a chronic fatigue syndrome. In many ways they have strengthened it while putting it in better perspective. It is currently felt that chronic Epstein-Barr virus infection does occur, but the most readily appreciated forms of that infection are rare and progressive in nature. In these disorders, active infection leads to inflammation in the lung, liver, and eye, and impairment of the production of blood cells by the bone marrow. In addition to fatigue there are intermittent high fevers, night sweats, weight loss, shortness of breath, and multiple abnormalities of blood chemistry.

This form of chronic Epstein-Barr virus infection is vastly different from the syndrome described by the Gregg Fishers of this world. Moreover, an illness like Gregg's is not a prelude to the progressive form of this disease. There is not sufficient evidence that active infection is occurring in the chronic fatigue syndrome. On the contrary, it is increasingly likely that the manifestations of the syndrome reflect an imbalance in the immune system.

There is no doubt that the chronic fatigue syndrome can follow Epstein-Barr virus–induced infectious mononucleosis, but only the minority of patients provide this history. We had thought for some time that even in the absence of a history of infectious mononucleosis, Epstein-Barr virus could often precipitate the syndrome. This was based upon the knowledge that first exposure to Epstein-Barr virus infection does not usually lead to a mononucleosis-like illness: the majority of initial infections are asymptomatic.

In contrast, we found that in most patients the chronic fatigue follows upper respiratory infections, hepatitis, gastrointestinal infections, or a variety of other infectious patterns not associated with Epstein-Barr virus. Additionally, there have been many outbreaks of similar chronic fatiguing illnesses reported for over a half century, a pattern of disease transmission that is not typical of Epstein-Barr virus. It is difficult to transmit Epstein-Barr virus. Furthermore, true epidemics of Epstein-Barr virus disease are rare. Finally, we have identified persons with the chronic fatigue syndrome who lack any antibodies to Epstein-Barr virus, indicating that they have never been infected by it.

Taken together, these observations teach us that other agents may be more important causes of the chronic fatigue syndrome.

What else could trigger the syndrome and how might it do so? The most likely causes include the viruses, ones that are well understood and possibly ones that are yet to be discovered. Viruses are remarkably diverse substances. They range in volume nearly a thousandfold. Some are very simple while others are complex, beginning to resemble the more sophisticated bacteria-like organisms. There are viruses that frequently cause fatal infections, and others which are not known to cause disease. Some viruses are cleared from the body by our immune defenses whereas others merely go into hiding and remain within us for life. Their evolutionary pattern is characterized by diverse strategies to infect us and to perpetuate themselves. How could a chronic illness have so many different causes? It is the solution to this dilemma that forces us to focus on ourselves as being part of the problem and the illness.

Our body possesses a complex network of defenses designed to ward off a myriad of incursions. There is not a different defense system for each infectious agent. Rather, the several elements of the immune system align themselves as needed to resist any of the thousands of different viruses, bacteria, fungi, and parasites. In the best of circumstances they defend us in a coordinated and balanced fashion; however, when the body's defenses are inadequate to the challenge of a virulent pathogen, disease results.

In other instances, the defenses may exceed what is required, and we inflict damage upon ourselves. For example, it is believed that the chemicals which mediate the responses necessary to clear foreign substances from our bodies induce inflammation, fever, and muscle aches. In mild cases such as respiratory infections, we feel sick all over, even though the infection is very localized. In extreme cases, components of the immune system can lead to inflammation and gradual destruction of blood vessels, joints, and other vital structures. So, too, may it be that the chronic fatigue syndrome results from the immune system's defense aimed initially at one of many infectious agents but eventually gone astray and directed persistently at ourselves.

As complex as this sounds, it may be all too naive, and much additional work is needed to begin to address this hypothesis. The current focus of research regarding this illness is multidisciplinary. Specialists in the fields of virology and immunology are working to isolate and characterize suspected infectious organisms that could either trigger or be responsible for the persistence of this syndrome. The field of immunology is developing further diagnostic tools for specificity in detecting alterations in the immune system. Clinicians are prospectively evaluating individuals affected by this illness in a collaborative fashion with specialists in virology, immunology, neuropsychology, psychiatry, and endocrinology. Such collective efforts are critical for a complete understanding of the underlying mechanisms responsible for this syndrome and in the subsequent development of therapeutic tools.

Whatever cause or causes are established eventually for this syndrome, we must consider it to reflect more than a proverbial battle between infectious substances and ourselves. The mechanistic approach to this disease fails to appreciate the degree to which the illness causes social and psychological upheaval.

While Gregg Fisher's assessment of the mechanisms that underlie his illness may be limited, he has richly described the impact of the disease upon himself, his wife, family, and friends. He must contend not only with frequent discomfort but, more importantly, also with uncertainty, dependence, and unfulfilled dreams.

Gregg Fisher's illness forced him to terminate his studies at the seminary. Thwarted from pursuing that profession in which he could guide and console coreligionists, he is relegated now to direct his truly limited energies to inform his fellow sufferers about this illness and to offer methods toward effective coping. This book is a testimony to the degree to which a man of certain faith remains optimistic and generous to those whose needs are no greater than his own.

EPILOGUE

It is difficult to try to put the finishing touches on a book about my illness when my illness has no finishing touches. This book is about my travail with CFS. It can never truly have an ending until my illness has an ending.

I pray that this ending comes soon, for all of us. Until that time does come, we are forced to place some of the best parts of our lives on hold. In a sense, each one of us is waiting to live, longing to exhilarate in what most others take for granted: good health. For living and health go hand in hand.

Though many of our highest hopes and brightest dreams are painfully beyond our grasp, we still must try to make the best of every day. Unfortunately, there is no easy way of making the best of CFS. I still struggle every day with my illness, and it never gets any easier. In fact, the most difficult chapter to write in this entire book was the one on coping. I felt hypocritical, knowing that there are not enough chapters in all the books in all the libraries of the world to make coping with this affliction truly easy. The best I could hope to do was bare a part of my soul, so that you could see there is someone else who knows what you are going through—to try to encourage you by sharing some of the ways I have learned to cope with my illness. When all is said and done, however, you are the only one who can cope with your illness; no one can do it for you. Others can help make the burden a little lighter, but it's still your burden.

There is a wonderfully moving anonymous poem entitled "Footprints in the Sand," about a man who dreams about his life. He sees two sets of footprints, one belonging to him and one belonging to God. He notices that during the lowest and saddest times in his life, there is only one set of footprints. Feeling betrayed and abandoned, he cries to God, "Lord, you said that once I decided to follow you, you'd walk with me all the way. But I have noticed that during the most troublesome times in my life, there is only one set of footprints. I don't understand why, when I needed you most, you would leave me." God replied, "My precious, precious child, I love you and I would never leave you. During those times of trial and suffering, when you saw only one set of footprints, it was then that I carried you."

Because of the faithfulness of God, the love of Shawn, and the support of family and friends, I have been carried through the trials of this illness more times than I can count. Till my dying day, I will never forget those who walked beside me, and for me, when I could not walk alone or at all.

Many images have been impressed upon my heart during the painfully long years of this affliction. The one that stands out most vividly is the precious spirit of one sick little boy. I don't know his name and I met him only briefly, but the impact he has had on my life has been profound.

I met this boy during one of our monthly hospital visits for gamma globulin treatments in Newark, New Jersey. CFS patients were treated in the pediatrics wing of the hospital, and, as was usually the case, there were too many patients that day and too few rooms. While Shawn and I were in the waiting room, an adorable little boy walked up to me. He was around five years old, with big brown eyes and a disarming smile. I do not know what disease he was suffering from because neither he nor his mother spoke English. We did share a common language though: the language of the sick.

He played make-believe doctor, and I was his patient. This little five-year-old was able to imitate hospital procedure flawlessly. In the world of imagination, he took my pulse, put a tourniquet around my upper arm and performed a blood test. Next, he unwrapped a make-believe IV needle and inserted it in my arm, in the right place and in the right direction. Then he started a make-believe IV pump. After the "treatment" was complete, he reversed the procedure, removing everything in the proper sequence. Finally, with obvious gentleness and concern, he placed a make-believe Band-Aid at the site where the IV needle had been.

My eyes filled with tears then, and do so again even as I write. Here was a little boy so obviously acquainted with pain and suffering that hospital procedures were indelibly imprinted on his little heart—a heart tiny in size, but filled with immense love. As he left with his mother to see his doctor, I couldn't help but picture everything he had just done to me in his make-believe world—this time happening in painful reality. I could imagine his little bottom lip quivering, with tears welling in his big brown eyes, as doctors treated him for a disease he could not comprehend—with needles and medications he could only perceive as hurtful, not helpful. Yet, through everything he had obviously suffered, his eyes had not the slightest hint of bitterness, resentment, or self-pity.

Whenever I start feeling sorry for myself, or bitter and resentful, I try to remember that little boy. For all of his short life he has known suffering, yet his spirit was as pure and gentle as any I have ever known. My highest aspiration is that my spirit may become as inspirational to others as that little boy's was to me. There is nothing about suffering that I don't loathe. But if I must suffer, I pray that it may make me a better person rather than a bitter one. My prayer for you is the same.

ACKNOWLEDGMENTS

A book is very rarely the product of one person. If this is true for healthy authors, it takes on a whole new meaning when the author is ill. This book has my name on it because it relates my struggle with CFS, but many people deserve to share the credit for writing it. I would especially like to thank Bernard Fisher, Caren Heacock, Mary Fisher, Ann Hibbard, and Donald Mulford for their assistance in writing, editing, rewriting, and typing the manuscript; Ed Sedarbaum for his insightful editing of this edition; and Charles Conrad and Warner Books for believing in this book.

I am indebted to Drs. Stephen E. Straus, Paul R. Cheney, James M. Oleske, and Irena Brus and to Janet Dale, R.N. for their editorial guidance and/or for contributing chapters, and to Themis Fotieo and Terence Linn for their legal counsel. While the advice these medical and legal professionals provided was invaluable, I alone am responsible for what I've written.

I would also like to express my gratitude to some of the many people who have lovingly given their support over the long years of this illness. To my precious wife, Shawn, who makes each day better than the one before and means more to me than she will ever know. To my parents, Mary and Bernard, whose sensitivity and love see me through every day. To Caren and Eric, and Aunt Dory and Uncle Ralph who are always there when we need them. To John Barlass, Lou Barlass, and Grandmother for caring and giving so much. To our special friends, Rita and Sam, Ken and Karen, Greg and Julie, Dave and Laura, Steve and Marta, Lynnie and Dave, Carolyn, Cynthia, Johnny and Betsy, Lucy and Bob. To the best friends I could ever hope for: Scotty, Roy and Betty, and Brenda. To Aunt Dorothy, Elfreide and the Voltmer cousins: Chris and Lauren, Ted and Barbie, Maryanna and John and Carrie, Paul, and Dorothea. To Darlene, Laurie, Dan and Barb, Scott, Grandma, and especially Mikaela, Joy, Charity, Jacob, and Faith, who have spent most of their little lives praying for us. To Bob, Sybil, Janet, Judy, Rich and Dar, and our other CFS friends. Special thanks to Dr. Berman, Dr. Matook, Dr. James, Dr. Pittman, Dr. Baker, Dr. Deutsch, and Peggy and Helen. To everyone at the Montclair Times, Nancy, Sara, Donna, Jerry, Wood Graphics, and Phyllis. To Gene and Lois, Dale and Terry (and M.J., too) for the healing waters. To Nana and Aunt Edna, gone but not forgotten. To Uncle Irv and Aunt Kaye, Claire, the Wynnes, Marilyn, Snappy, Bob, Chris, the Olsens, Hy Cohen, Calvary Evangelical Free Church, and Mattituck Presbyterian Church. Thanks to all those who have been praying for us. Finally, I want to give all glory and honor to God, who makes life worth living no matter what the circumstances.

APPENDIX A
Gregg Fisher's Doctor
Talks to Yours

What follows is a memo written by my doctor, James M. Oleske, for physicians of patients complaining of chronic fatigue syndrome. If your physician hasn't had much experience with CFS, you might want to share this memo with him.

9 May 1988

Since 1980, two new diseases have made an impact on the health of our patients and have stressed the medical care system. The most obvious and lethal has been human immunodeficiency virus (HIV) infection and AIDS. Somewhat overshadowed but still disabling both physically and mentally has been chronic fatigue syndrome (CFS), also known as chronic Epstein-Barr virus infection (CEBV).

These latter patients have a confusing illness, the hallmark of which is disabling fatigue over long periods of time. Complicating this syndrome are a variety of other symptoms related to chronic encephalopathy, arthralgia, gastrointestinal upset, recurrent pharyngitis, and cervical adenopathy.

As confusing as the individual symptoms are to the physician, so are the usual lack of collaborating physical findings and diagnostic laboratory studies. Frustration and secondary depression are frequent components to the patient who has already seen a number of general physicians as well as specialists. Many physician encounters with such patients consist of an all-too-brief history, curtailed physical exam, and limited laboratory evaluation. The diagnostic outcome is predictable. The patient is diagnosed as depressed, as psychosomatic, or as a malingerer. Because of the limited number of medically sound studies of CFS, the evaluating physician has little literature on which to base a specific diagnosis. There are several scientifically sound studies now under way examining the question of CFS. Publication of studies on epidemiology, natural history, etiopathogenesis, and therapy trials will, in time, define the parameters of this syndrome so that patients may be more appropriately evaluated, diagnosed, and treated. In the meantime, since 1976, I have had experience in evaluating over one hundred children and adults with severe mononucleosis syndrome and/or chronic fatigue.

Patients with EBV acute mononucleosis are frequently adolescents or young adults. This acute viral infection with EBV is now well described. There is, however, a lack of appreciation as to how severe and prolonged a bout of EBV mononucleosis may be for an individual patient. Some patients may have persistence of symptoms, especially fatigue, for one to two years after a severe bout of acute EBV infectious mononucleosis (IM). Rarely have I seen adolescent patients who have experienced periodic flare-ups of sore throat, cervical adenopathy, and fatigue two to four years after the initial bout of acute IM. In general, however, such adolescent and young adult patients completely recover and do not progress to what has been called CFS or CEBV syndrome. Only a longer period of observation of such patients, however, will answer the question of the relationship of severity of acute IM and the development later in life of CFS.

The recently appreciated CFS usually occurs in young adults, females more frequently than males. In our group of eighty patients, the mean age was 28 years with a range of 12–50 years. There was a female-to-male ratio of cases of 2:1. The accompanying table lists the signs and symptoms we have seen in our group of patients. The *Annals of Internal Medicine* published a clinical case definition for CFS in May 1988.

In general, patients with CFS give a history of past acute IM, but usually several years in the past, with an intervening history of good health. The first bout of CFS usually begins as a flulike illness from which the patient never completely recovers. Patients may have continuous symptoms that are made worse by intercurrent illness, or emotional or physical stress. Other patients have episodes of symptoms that may last for one to six weeks interspersed with some periods of relative well-being. During a flare-up of symptoms, the patient usually is so fatigued he or she can perform no useful tasks. The major symptoms appear related to CNS dysfunction, a flulike illness with arthralgia and GI upset. A general pattern that I have seen is an initial flu illness that becomes progressively worse, with fatigue and other symptoms, which peaks in severity at one to three years. Thereafter, there is gradual improvement in symptoms over the next two to ten years. The true course of recovery varies greatly from patient to patient. There are frequent exacerbations of symptoms during which patients feel they are again as sick as before. However, when patients more objectively evaluate their symptoms, there is slow, gradual recovery of CFS for most patients. I have not seen, nor has the medical literature reported, an increased incidence of malignancy in patients with CFS. I have cared for eight women with CFS who have become pregnant and have had completely normal infants. Most of these women had uneventful pregnancies, and many reported an improvement in their CFS during pregnancy. None of these women have shown worsening of the CFS postpartum.

Based on a review of the literature and my own experience, I would urge the physician presented with a patient with complaints of chronic fatigue to consider the following guidelines in their medical evaluation and care.

1. Allow enough time for an adequate history (at least a half hour), and prior to the initial patient visit, make every attempt to obtain any previous medical records. Many patients with CFS have seen health care providers before they are seen by you. The initial encounters with the physician for the patient with CFS should be devoted to differential diagnosis to ensure that the suspected CFS patient's multiple complaints are not due to other causes (i.e., multiple sclerosis, inflammatory bowel disease, collagen vascular disease, Lyme disease, hepatitis [A, B, and Non-A, Non-B], chronic asthma, adult onset of cystic fibrosis, allergies, HIV infection, unusual infections like brucellosis, SBE, tuberculosis, lymphoma, or Behçet's syndrome). The workup for these diverse diseases needs to be selected laboratory studies guided by a thorough history and careful physical exam. At the very least, patients with suspected CFS should have a CBC differential and platelet count, sed rate, multiple blood chemistry, ANA, C3/C4/CH50, U/A, and chest X ray. If there are episodes of fever, patients should also have several blood cultures taken and, if GI symptoms are present, stools examined for O & P as well as cultured. A more aggressive FUO evaluation will need to be considered in patients with persistent episodes of fever. Patients with predominant CNS symptomatology suggesting a chronic encephalopathy (confusion, episodes of lack of concentration, headache, depression, insomnia) may benefit from a more detailed neurological evaluation by a consultant neurologist.

2. The more specific assay to evaluate the suspected CFS patient will also include EBV titers that examine for VCA-IgG, early antigen (restricted and diffuse), and EBNA titers. Because of my experience with humoral immune deficiency in patients with CFS, I also would recommend that such patients have quantitative immunoglobulin (IgG, A, M, E) and IgG subclass levels performed. If these humoral immune studies are abnormal, such patients probably should be referred to an immunologist for further immune system evaluation.

3. There is no specific diagnostic test for CFS although some patterns of laboratory abnormalities tend to support an organic basis for the patient with CFS. Since it is not proven, but suspected by some, that CFS may be caused by Epstein-Barr virus, the serial prospective evaluation of EBV titers may be helpful in some cases. Other viral and noninfective cases of CFS will obviously not be reflected in EBV titers. The finding of persistently high VCA-IgG with higher early antigen titer than EBNA titers is the most characteristic finding described in the literature. A patient, however, may have CFS with other patterns of EBV titers. In 20 percent of patients I have seen, besides high EBV titers there are markedly increased CMV titers. In 40 percent of cases I have evaluated for CFS, there have been noted low/normal total IgG levels and low IgG subclass levels. The finding of persistently elevated EBV titers and IgG subclass deficiency is strong evidence that an individual patient has CFS based on chronic viral (EBV) infection. The diagnosis of CFS, however, is usually one of exclusion and only partially supported by laboratory studies presently available.

4. One role the physician caring for a patient with suspected CFS must include is advocacy. While recognizing that the physician must evaluate and suspect emotional/psychological illness and make appropriate referrals, many patients with CFS are suffering from a poorly understood organic syndrome probably related to a persistent viral infection. Many of such patients' emotional distresses and depression are related to their chronic illness and frequent disbelief by their physicians, friends, and family. Even if most CFS patients were suffering from a psychosomatic illness (I do not believe this to be the case), they still deserve the care and compassion of their private physican. They should not be simply told to go elsewhere because a physician cannot make a specific diagnosis. It is the role of a primary care physician to adequately evaluate such patients, offer supportive care that is appropriate and without harm, and help their patients with a chronic illness avoid being victimized by "fringe" health care providers. Constant referrals to multiple specialists are usually not helpful to the patient or primary care doctor, especially if a careful initial evaluation is performed.

5. There is no specific therapy for CFS. Antiviral trials with acyclovir (directed against EBV) have not been demonstrated to be effective and have some potential to cause harm (e.g., renal disease). Symptomatic care and emotional support are important in improving the life-style and condition of an individual with CFS. The best individual to coordinate this program would be a nonjudgmental and committed primary care physician. CFS patients usually do poorly when they receive care from a number of subspecialists. Any patient with a chronic illness needs emotional support to manage the stress of his or her illness. Many patients with CFS would benefit from the techniques available through a psychologist (i.e., stress management, self-hypnosis, behavior modification, etc.). Only infrequently do such patients require referral to a psychiatrist.

As with any chronic illness, good nutrition is important, but CFS is not caused by a vitamin/mineral deficiency. A daily vitamin/mineral supplement is a reasonable recommendation, but megavitamin therapy is not. Patients do benefit from limited exercise that gives a psychological lift but is not so strenuous that it results in a relapse of more severe fatigue. Patients with CFS seem to have a greater risk of having exacerbation or onset of typical allergic diseases with onset of their CFS. Such individuals with asthma, rhinitis, conjunctivitis, and other inhalant allergic symptoms should receive appropriate allergic care, which may include the use of Seldane 60 mg BID or TID. This antihistamine does not cross the blood-brain barrier and therefore does not exacerbate the fatigue as is the tendency of other antihistamines. Other allergic therapies and evaluation may be helpful depending on the individual's specific symptoms. Many of the patients I have seen with CFS have insomnia or poor sleep habits despite feeling exhausted. Such patients may benefit from taking a tricyclic antidepressant before bedtime. I have used Sinequan 10–75 mg at night for thirty CFS patients and over half felt marked improvement. Appropriate care, however, must be exercised in the use of these medications.

When headache is a major manifestation of a CFS patient, I have tried therapy with Diamox 500 mg sequels taken at bedtime. This mild diuretic possibly lowers CSF pressure as it does in decreasing anterior eye chamber pressure in glaucoma. Some patients complain of "tingling" in their hands with Diamox. Of twenty-five patients I have treated with Diamox, fifteen had improved after a two-week daily course and I have maintained them on dose schedules of two to three times per week with no significant side effects and continued improvement in headache symptoms.

The frequent joint symptoms and generalized aches and pains that many patients with CFS experience with an exacerbation will sometimes be improved with a nonsteroidal anti-inflammatory agent. I have had personal success with Feldene 20 mg daily in several of my patients, but I doubt there is any advantage to this agent over other, similar medications. The use of steroids in CFS is very controversial, and the serious side effects and toxicity of this hormone must always be remembered. Only infrequently would the risks of using steroids be outweighed by possible benefits in a specific patient. There are indications for steroids in acute EBV mononucleosis syndrome (impending upper airway obstruction, impending rupture of the spleen, cardiomyopathy, encephalitis, and severe hemolytic anemia). The patient with acute IM treated with steroids often has dramatic improvement including a feeling of well-being and a lessening of fatigue. However, the long-term risk of using steroids with a known latent viral agent having oncogenic potential is a major therapeutic decision requiring careful evaluation of benefit and risk. Likewise for the patient with a chronic illness, such as CFS (possibly the result of uncontrolled expression of EBV), the use of steroids has significant theoretical risks and little proven benefit. While considering the above, there have been rare circumstances when I have given a course of prednisone to a patient with CFS. The use of steroids in such cases may provide a short period of relief of symptoms, but the long-term use of prednisone even in a low-dose, alternate-day schedule should not be recommended.

When a patient with CFS is identified to have an antibody deficiency, replacement therapy with intravenous gamma globulin needs to be considered. Approximately 40 percent of patients I have seen with CFS have low/normal IgG and IgG subclass deficiency. This group of patients when treated with IV gamma globulin has had symptomatic improvements with less fatigue, sore throats, and cervical adenopathy. The cost of IV gamma globulin is significant ($1000/month), and this limits its use to those patients with defined antibody deficiency associated with their CFS.

Other symptomatic therapies include management of the frequent GI disturbance seen in such patients, and occasional referrals to a gastrointestinal specialist are part of the care required by CFS patients. As the syndrome of CFS becomes defined and *appreciated*, appropriate patient referral to research centers may yield a specific causative agent or agents. Once the etiopathogenesis can be defined, diagnostic laboratory criteria will be established. The lack of a specific etiology, however, should not exclude the development of controlled treatment trials for some of the therapies outlined. Specifically, tricyclic antidepressants, Diamox, and IV gamma globulin should be therapies that are evaluated in controlled studies of CFS patients.

Despite the lack of specific diagnostic tests, the physician who has a patient with suspected CFS seeking his or her help and care should respond with compassion while performing the workup previously outlined. During the several weeks and visits such an evaluation will require to make this diagnosis of exclusion, the primary care physician should provide emotional and symptomatic care. If, after an appropriate workup and period of observation, the physician is convinced that a patient has a nonorganic psychological process, then he should make the appropriate referrals for the best care of his patient. However, if after such a workup a patient appears to have CFS, the primary care physician should continue to supervise the care of his patient, including coordinating the input from any subspecialists seen by the patient.

The primary care physician should help his patients with CFS negotiate the difficult problems they will encounter with entitlement programs and insurance companies. Those patients who are disabled and unable to work need to have their physician provide supported documentation to Social Security.

It is inappropriate for physicians to claim they "don't believe" patients can have chronic fatigue syndrome. The physician needs to evaluate each patient thoroughly and carefully. Whether the patients with disabling chronic fatigue symptoms suffer from an as-yet poorly understood organic process or a psychosomatic illness, they deserve to have a physician who will provide compassionate care, appreciated advice, and referral, while maintaining patient contact and advocacy.

CLINICAL SIGNS AND SYMPTOMS IN
80 CFS PATIENTS

Fatigability	(80)	100%
Depression	(73)	91%
Body weakness	(70)	87%
Headache	(57)	71%
Decreased concentration/memory	(52)	65%
Glandular swelling (L.N.)	(52)	65%
School/job failure	(50)	63%
Fever	(42)	52%
Sore throat	(42)	52%
Abdominal pain/cramps	(34)	43%
Arthralgia/stiff joints	(33)	41%
Allergy-like symptoms	(28)	35%
Body aches/myalgia	(28)	35%
Confusion	(21)	26%
Lethargy	(21)	26%
Rash	(14)	17%
Puffy eyelids	(14)	17%
Nausea	(14)	17%
Hepatosplenomegaly	(14)	17%
Blurring vision/photophobia	(10)	13%
Dizziness	(10)	13%
Swelling hands	(9)	11%
Vomiting	(9)	11%
Diarrhea	(7)	9%
Shortness of breath	(7)	9%
Suicidal attempt	(3)	4%
Clumsiness	(3)	4%
Hair loss	(3)	4%
Hallucination	(3)	4%
Raynaud's phenomenon	(2)	2%
Recurrent aseptic meningitis	(2)	2%
Slurred speech	(2)	2%
Tinnitus	(2)	2%
Loss of taste and smell	(2)	2%

APPENDIX B
CFS Research: Questions, Challenges, and Obstacles
by Paul R. Cheney, M.D., Ph.D., Senior Staff Physician, Nalle Clinic, Charlotte, North Carolina

Chronic fatigue syndrome (CFS) relates to a chronic, relapsing, and often evolving illness usually characterized by dysfunctional fatigue, recurrent pharyngitis, adenopathy, headache, low-grade fever, muscle and joint aches, cognitive disorders, and neuropsychiatric problems. Chronic fatigue and immunodysfunction syndrome (CFIDS) relates to that subcategory of CFS patients for whom objective evidence exists of significant immune dysfunction or perturbation. Whether these "abnormal findings" represent a primary immunologic defect resulting in loss of control of certain ubiquitous but usually latent viral infections, or are secondary to chronic active infection by an immunotropic virus, or are secondary to some other process cannot at present be determined with confidence. It is highly likely that these situations can exist separately but vicious cycles may be set up that make it difficult to determine the exact causal agent or mechanism. The almost inevitable influence of cofactors, both endogenous (i.e., genetic or developmental) and exogenous (i.e., environmental or coinfections), makes this one of the most challenging disorders ever studied. Threads of new insight weave their way from CFS into a host of other medical conditions, both well defined and poorly defined. To study this disorder is in a sense to study a much larger part of medicine because many of the same elements can be seen in other diseases due to common physiologic and pathophysiologic pathways. However, the fact that CFS has erupted onto the medical landscape as a reasonably common, clinically recognizable condition that may also be on the rise raises an important question. Is there some new agent or factor driving most cases of CFS/CFIDS that have developed in the last ten or fifteen years?

Because of the usually abrupt onset and mono-like clinical character as well as the serologic findings of increased Epstein-Barr virus (EBV) replication activity, this illness quickly assumed in the United States the label "chronic Epstein-Barr virus syndrome" (CEBV) or "chronic mononucleosis syndrome." In a substantial number of patients, however, evidence of abnormal EBV activity is lacking and a few patients with this syndrome are sero-negative for EBV. Despite lack of EBV ubiquity, which challenges its role as a cause of the syndrome, the Epstein-Barr virus will likely always be associated with this syndrome either as a secondary effect in most cases or as a primary cause of disease in an important but undetermined minority of these patients.

Recently, there has been a growing impression that CFS is increasing in frequency in the population. The syndrome may be well represented in the 20 percent of primary care patients who complain of significant and prolonged fatigue of abrupt onset. Half of all patients given the diagnosis of fibromyalgia may find the label CFS a better fit. Outbreaks of this syndrome have been reported and strongly suggest that a novel agent or set of factors is at play in a virgin population. Indeed, the best candidate as a novel cause of CFS is the newly discovered human herpesvirus 6 or HHV6. The apparent laboratory behavior of HHV6 could, if present in this condition, allow it to eclipse EBV as an associated if not causal factor in CFS. There may well be other undiscovered infectious agents and cofactors that could combine to make this a true "witches' brew" of a problem. It is even possible that no single or group of infectious agents is primarily responsible but that these agents are secondary effects of an environmental immunotoxin. Beyond infectious agents and toxins lies the concept of stress. While stress can play a role in any disease, it may play a far more central role in CFS. Stress can clearly modulate the cycles of symptoms, promote relapse of symptoms, and is often implicated at the onset of this syndrome. The relationship of stress to CFS is clear enough to suggest it as a cofactor but probably not the cause of CFS. Too many patients have little or no stress involved at the onset or relapse of their symptoms.

Despite the increasing weight of evidence that this syndrome is a real disease with measurable immunologic, serologic, and neurologic abnormalities, many institutions and prominent physicians scoff at this problem and the patients who have it. It is therefore important to move quickly to establish ever-more objective markers for this syndrome and to search out its basic pathophysiology and ideally its cause(s). Quite apart from the professional divisions over this syndrome, this could be a very serious and widespread health problem.

Probably the most important question about CFS is whether or not its frequency is increasing and, if so, why? Chronic fatigue syndrome is clearly related to several vaguely defined syndromes, both epidemic and sporatic, described in the medical literature since the late nineteenth century. The concept of a postviral fatigue syndrome is likely to be a valid clinical entity as old as viruses and man. Postviral neuromyasthenia, as it was called by some in the older medical literature, seemingly was either common or prolonged but not both. Postviral fatigue in its common form was self-limited and only rarely was it prolonged. If epidemic, then it was geographically confined to a small locality and never generalized to an entire nation. CFS, as defined in the opening paragraph, now appears to be both common, prolonged, epidemic, and generalized across national boundaries, which suggests an immediate difference with past descriptions. An apparent rise in cases, probably from the

1970s, both in this country and overseas, suggests a pandemic. Random national surveys by this author of groups of patients who joined CEBV support groups in 1986 show an exponential case production curve beginning in the early to mid-1970s with 70 percent of patients becoming ill in the last five years. The fidelity of this survey data from region to region, as well as the rate of rise established well before media interest began in 1985–86, argues in favor of its validity. If valid then there may be more than one interpretation, including the possibility that CFS is about five years in length for most patients, which would produce a similar curve to the one observed. At the moment no one can know the truth with certainty. One possibility may be that a new agent is creating a pandemic of CFS since the early 1970s, superimposed on a constant baseline production of similar-appearing cases of postviral fatigue syndrome. Postviral fatigue, or neuromyasthenia, then represents a much older, and probably generic problem. What is more farfetched than this view is that we could have, in the closing years of the twentieth century, such a poor clinical concept of an "old" disease that is as common and impressive as CFS is today. How could we have missed this often impressive disorder for so long? Today's CFS patients can easily write books on a disorder that has generated only a handful of research papers in a hundred years. Too many good clinicians have stated, "I've never seen anything quite like this," and perhaps they are right.

Another important question concerns how to make the diagnosis of CFS/CFIDS. When considering a diagnosis of CFS, one is often faced with a group of alternate diagnoses, the so-called differential diagnoses. A recent publication has given a rather extensive list of other possibilities that, while possible in a given case, have not proven to be very commonly found in the experience of most referral clinicians who deal with CFS. That so few patients have been found to have "other, more plausible explanations" for their symptoms is remarkable and attests to the validity of CFS as a clinical entity. There are, however, several related disorders that are most often considered and that may not, for a variety of reasons, be easily dismissed. In order of frequency they are:

1. Depression or related mood disorders
2. Somatization disorder
3. Fibromyalgia
4. Constitutional deficit since childhood/adolescence
5. Allergies and other sensitivities
6. Multiple sclerosis
7. Neuromuscular disorders of uncertain cause
8. Acute infectious mono with prolonged recovery
9. Autoimmune disorders

The relationship of CFS to the above disorders may be closer than the usual list of differential diagnoses. Many patients given a diagnosis from the above list are just CFS patients by another name or vice versa. It is likely that similar pathophysiologic mechanisms are at work to explain some of the symptom similarities. There may also be genetic and other factors that predispose people to disorders that possess related pathophysiologies. Finally, it is possible that CFS itself can produce in some patients a clinical picture identical to some of the above diagnoses. Despite the admittedly complex relationship of CFS to the above disorders, the usual case of CFS can be differentiated on clinical and other grounds and may have unique and, more recently, even novel causes.

Serious obstacles to further progress are lack of a consensus over case definition and political divisions in our medical research centers over whether this problem even exists. Lack of a good case definition will quickly lead to studies of "fatigue" patients with too heterogeneous a mix of pathophysiologies to give meaningful results. A lack of coherent and reproducible studies will only fuel professional divisions. Another problem is the relative lack of rigorous and systematic clinical database collections on a large group of these patients in one place who can be followed over time. Longitudinal clinical studies will help determine separate subpopulations of these patients. Analysis of subpopulations will be very important if patients who meet a given case definition are ill from different agents or pathophysiologic mechanisms. It is possible, however, that a case definition exists in which the great majority of patients are ill from a single agent or basic mechanism. As discussed above, it is almost certain that several pathophysiologic mechanisms exist in CFS that also operate in many other diseases. Insights gained from the study of CFS will likely have "spin-offs" for a number of other both organic and apparently psychiatric disorders often equated or associated with CFS.

APPENDIX C
Where To Go For Help

The following CFS organizations are the largest in the country. They publish newsletters and can help you find a local support group in your general area.

Chronic Fatigue Syndrome Association
919 Scott Avenue
Kansas City, Kansas 66105
(913) 321-2278

Chronic Fatigue Immune Dysfunction Society Association
Community Health Services
1401 East Seventh Street
Charlotte, North Carolina 28204
(704) 375-0172

Chronic Fatigue Syndrome Society
P.O. Box 230108
Portland, Oregon 97223
(503) 684-5261

The Lung Line is a toll free number established by the National Jewish Center for Immunology and Respiratory Medicine in Denver, Colorado, to answer questions about CFS.

(800) 222-5864 (LUNG)

The Centers for Disease Control and the National Institutes of Health send free CFS information packets upon request.

Centers for Disease Control
Attn. Josephine Lister
Bldg. 6 Room 121
Atlanta, Georgia 30333
(404) 639-1338

**National Institute of Allergy
and Infectious Diseases**
Office of Communications
Bldg. 31 Room 7A-32
Bethesda, Maryland 20892

The CFS Research Foundation is a nonprofit corporation formed to raise money for CFS research.

CFS Research Foundation
c/o National Jewish Center for
Immunology and Respiratory Medicine
P.O. Box 6747
Denver, Colorado 80206

Minann, a nonprofit foundation which has dedicated itself to medical and educational matters, promotes public awareness and funding for CFS research.

Minaan, INC.
P.O. Box 582
Glenview, Illinois 60025

The following organizations provide information on CFS research and support groups outside of the U.S.:

A.N.Z.M.E. Society
P.O. Box 35-429, Browns Bay
Aukland 10, New Zealand

Myalgic Encephalomyelitis Association
P.O. Box 8
Stanford le Hope 8EL
Essex SS17 8EX England

APPENDIX D
Further Reading

GENERAL

Jeffreys, Toni. *The Mile-High Staircase*. Auckland London Sydney: Hodder & Stoughton, 1982.

Johnson, Hillary. "Journey Into Fear: The Growing Nightmare of Epstein-Barr Virus." *Rolling Stone* 504/505 (July 16, 1987): 54, 506 (August 13, 1987): 42.

Kleimann, Leanne. "Yuppie Flu: Do You Have It?" *Health* (April 1988): 64.

Marsa, Linda. "Newest Mystery Illness: Chronic Fatigue Syndrome." *Redbook* 170 (April 1988): 120.

National Institute of Allergy and Infectious Diseases. National Institutes of Health. Office of Communication. "Backgrounder: Chronic Fatigue Syndrome." Bethesda, Maryland, June 1988.

Podell, Richard N. *Doctor, Why Am I So Tired?* New York: Pharos, 1988.

Stoff, Jesse A. and Charles R. Pellegrino. *Chronic Fatigue Syndrome: The Hidden Epidemic*. New York: Random House, 1988.

TECHNICAL

Buchwald, Dedra. John L. Sullivan. Anthony L. Komaroff. "Frequency of 'Chronic Active Epstein-Barr Virus Infection' in a General Medical Practice." *JAMA* 257 (May 1, 1987): 2303-2307.

Grierson, Helen, et al. "Coping With Chronic Fatigue Syndrome." *Patient Care* 21 (Nov. 15, 1987): 79.

Holmes, Gary P., et al. "A Cluster of Patients With a Chronic Mononucleosis-like Syndrome." *JAMA* 257 (May 1, 1987): 2297-2302.

——————. "Chronic Fatigue Syndrome: A Working Case Definition." *Annals of Internal Medicine* 108 (March 1988): 387-389.

Jones, J.F., et al. "Evidence for Active Epstein-Barr Virus Infection in Patients With Persistent Unexplained Illnesses: Elevated Anti-Early Antigen Antibodies." *Annals of Internal Medicine* 102 (1985):1-7.

Smith, Douglas M. "Social Security Disability Assessment: Inseparable From Patient Care." *Internal Medicine for the Specialist* 9 (1988): 51-63.

Straus, Stephen E. "The Chronic Mononucleosis Syndrome." *The Journal of Infectious Diseases* 157 (March 1988): 405-412.

——————. "EB or not EB: That is the Question." *JAMA* 257 (May 1, 1987): 2335.

Straus, Stephen E., et al. "Persisting Illness and Fatigue in Adults With Evidence of Epstein-Barr Virus Infection." *Annals of Internal Medicine* 102 (1985): 7-16.

INDEX